CHI
RUNNING

A REVOLUTIONARY APPROACH TO EFFORTLESS, INJURY-FREE RUNNING

Revised and Fully Updated

DANNY DREYER
AND KATHERINE DREYER

AUTHORS OF *CHIWALKING*

PRAISE FOR CHIRUNNING

"I have been running great thanks to ChiRunning. I continue to improve my technique and have easily cut 90 seconds per mile of my normal pace. It has helped me tremendously in the triathlon. Thanks again; I have told many other runners about ChiRunning. It's a great thing." —Todd Toriscelli, M.A., A.T.C.; head athletic trainer, Tampa Bay Buccaneers, age 42

"Running is an unusual sport. Most people taking up a sport such as tennis or golf have at some point obtained some lessons. Almost every recreational runner just runs, never having received any tips or instruction on form. I strongly feel that this book would allow tens of thousands of runners like myself to enjoy running without being injured. I found your principles extremely easy to adapt, and began running with minimal radicular pain, despite training vigorously on hills. Also, as you predicted, my overall energy expenditure for each run was considerably less than what I was used to."
—Tony Cucuzzella, M.D.

"As yoga teacher in residence and wellness director for the New York Road Runners, I have seen how stiff, tight, and injured runners can become when they think performance is simply about building leg strength and running more miles. Danny Dreyer's insightful approach can change all that. His remarkable program offers a completely new way to run without effort or injury."
—Beryl Bender Birch, author of *Power Yoga*

"I am rarely jolted by today's sports literature, but reading *ChiRunning,* I was thoroughly entranced by the vast wealth of information packed into it. When I realized that on every single page I was making notes of matters crucial to improving my running, I knew I had stumbled upon the most exciting and revolutionary book to hit the running community this decade. It will have you jumping from your seat to discover secrets that will, I believe, perfect and enrich your running experience."
—Toby Tanser, sub-2:20 marathoner; author of *Train Hard, Win Easy;* coach; member, New York Road Runners board of directors

"As a national-class runner, trained by some of the nation's top coaches, I doubted Danny would have much to offer that I didn't already know. Fortunately for my teams, as well as my own running, I kept an open mind. ChiRunning not only helped my level 1, 2, and 3 runners but it improved my running as well! His running technique improves performance at all levels and, most important, prevents injuries."

—April Powers, senior head marathon and triathlon coach, Team in Training; inner Madrid Marathon '83; Olympic Marathon Trials '84; silver medalist in Duathlon World Championships, Spain 1997; Wildflower Ironman age group champion '97

"The best thing about ChiRunning is that it makes so much sense! The principle of working with your core strength is very powerful and natural. This program will totally revolutionize the way you run."   —Baron Baptiste, author of *Journey into Power*

"This book makes running possible for everyone. The magical, concrete guidelines will educate and inspire your every footfall henceforth. Your running will be like play—all energy and no effort. Treat yourself, buy this book *now*, and run safely for as long as you like. It's just plain fun to read and the single most useful thing I have ever read about running. Bravo!"

—Jean Couch, director, Balance Center, Palo Alto; author of *The Runner's Yoga Book*

"ChiRunning is both spectacularly simple and unique. Danny Dreyer revolutionizes the sport by synthesizing running, T'ai Chi Chuan, and applied physics, inventing a new way to run that builds on ancient wisdom. Like the soft and supple power of water to cut through a mountain, he enables runners to propel themselves with less effort, improve their gait, increase their endurance, and knock their socks off by having a really good time."

—Harriet Beinfield and Efrem Korngold, coauthors, *Between Heaven and Earth: A Guide to Chinese Medicine*

"Danny Dreyer and ChiRunning gave me a precious gift. After being unable to run for ten years because of injury, at age 52 I'm again enjoying pleasurable, injury-free trail runs in the Shawangunk Mountains. I can now move on land with the same economy, flow, and mindfulness that make swimming such bliss for me. I tell people that *ChiRunning* is an owner's manual for anyone who has legs and the desire to use them for health and happiness."

—Terry Laughlin, author, *Total Immersion*

"After being unable to run for five years due to a back injury, ChiRunning helped get me back on the road. I highly recommend it for anyone who wants to run without injury."

—Jack Nelligan, M.D., orthopedic surgeon; former
400M record holder, Stanford University

"ChiRunning is a great way to practice the principles of Pilates while running. Danny's ChiRunning technique results in fluid movement working from your center. Using only the muscle work you need to be using and letting gravity be your friend lead to efficient movement, one of the key principles of Pilates! ChiRunning and Pilates are totally complementary! I highly recommend Danny's clear explanation of these healthy running concepts. Enjoy in great health."

—Sandra Sweet, owner of the Pilates/movement
education studio Feel Good Fitness

"Here we have another fine contribution to the awareness of the Tao in sports. This book is in tune with the Taoist wisdom of Wei Wu Wei—Doing Without Doing, to find true joy in the discipline of effortless running as a Way of Being."

—Chungliang Al Huang, president, Living Tao Foundation;
coauthor of *Thinking Body, Dancing Mind;* author of
Embrace Tiger, Return to Mountain, and *Tai Ji*

"After 21 years as a sports podiatrist specializing in running injuries and thousands of exams a year, I thought I had seen it all. Then a patient came in who, after taking a ChiRunning class, looked like a different runner—an amazing improvement. It was obvious his impact forces were minimized. Since then I have referred many happy patients to ChiRunning. This technique works to reduce injury, and with it virtually any runner can improve."

—David R. Hannaford, M.D., podiatrist

"Danny Dreyer has combined the practice of running with the philosophy of chi in a beautiful way. People who follow his method will enjoy a more stress-free and graceful way of running and living."
—Marilyn Tam, author of *How to Use What You've Got to Get What You Want*; former president, Reebok Apparel and Retail Group

"In our Learn to Run, Save a Life training program, ChiRunning has been exceptional. Beginning and experienced runners benefit from the emphasis on injury prevention through efficient biomechanics."
—Jeff Shapiro, M.D.; executive director, Organs 'R' Us; race director, Providian Relay (America's second largest relay)

"There are many things that distinguish great athletes like Tiger Woods, Barry Bonds, or Paula Radcliffe. They have all learned the axiom that less is more. And they had great mentors. Through this book, Danny Dreyer will become your coach and mentor. He will hand you the keys to a superior running experience. Danny is one of the most generous and talented coaches I know. If you cannot train with him personally, this book is the next best thing."
—David Deigan, coach emeritus, San Francisco Road Runners Club; CEO of AFM, Inc.; distance runner with over 45 years of experience

"I wanted to let you know that today was the first time I was able to fully apply the ChiRunning techniques. I was really amazed at how relaxed and strong I felt throughout the run. I wasn't looking forward to the end of the run and felt completely energized. When I passed another runner my heart smiled because I felt like I possessed a pretty potent secret weapon."
—Rick Muhr, regional coach, Team in Training, Boston

"From the single clinic I did with you I have grown immensely. Through what I learned in your clinic, I am in essence learning to walk again, and learning to run again, and the new ease I am finding there is continuing to spill over into all other aspects of my life."
—Darryl Denton, age 54, San Jose, California

"I've read and reread this book and am running like I've never run in my 42 years of running. To me, this is nothing short of a miracle! I'm also thinking about marathon running, something I'd never considered possible before! Chirunning has had a radical change on not just my running, but my overall fitness and physical feeling during the workday. I've bought multiple copies for family members who are avid runners and they're achieving similar results. Thank you, thank you, thank you for this book. It's nothing short of magical!"

—Dr. Mark O'Donnell, age 59

"Thank you for a life-changing book and DVD. I have benefited greatly from your program, and it has changed my life. I used to hate, hate, hate running and only put up with it because I loved, loved, loved triathlon (at least the biking and swimming parts). So I really appreciate the fact that I look forward to every run now, which is a wonderful blessing."

—Dean Carpenter

"I have an absolute passion for encouraging and supporting senior-age runners. I hope to run forever! 64 is the new 46 and I'm living proof. Life is *good*. Thanks again for your work, your expertise, your clear instruction, and your encouragement."

—Dr. Paul Timm, age 64

"I am a certified athletic trainer and have worked for over 13 years providing emergency medical and orthopedic injury care to collegiate athletes. And do I have to say it? My athletes will be the beneficiaries of Danny's wisdom in my everyday work life, with these principles turning their frustration into successes with simple instructions that they can easily absorb and immediately apply. As I reach my fiftieth birthday this spring, I know I will be out running and feeling like myself again—and a busload of athletes I know will be having *way* more fun."

—Dale Robinson-Gervais, A.T.C., age 50

"I have *never* written a testimonial in my life, and I really prefer to deflect attention. I am running faster than I ever have run in my life, setting PRs over the last year in virtually every distance. After many years, I have realized a dream of qualifying for Boston 2008, and I only feel I will improve. Most important, I'm running injury free. Thank you for having the courage to follow your dream and for sharing your discovery with the world."

—Randy Hunt, age 45

"I took your three-session class back in July. After the second session, I ran in the San Francisco Half Marathon and set a personal record by taking 9 minutes off my previous best time. Over the rest of the summer I recovered from some minor knee pain and I've been able to stop wearing the knee support straps I'd been using. I then entered the Silicon Valley Marathon. Using the techniques I gained from your class I was able to run the entire race without taking walking breaks and I completed the distance, taking a whopping 40 minutes off my previous best time!"   —Terry Ridgway, age 36, San Jose, California

"I have taken Danny Dreyer's running classes, and they are truly revolutionary. I've been a runner for more than forty years. In my mid-fifties I had knee surgery and was about to give it up. My body just couldn't take the punishment anymore.

"Then I took Danny's workshop and running is a joy again. Despite widespread information in the media about how arthritis in the knees and pain in the lower back is inevitable as we get older, Danny has simply proven them wrong. I'm now running much longer distances than ever, running up steep, long hills, and turning in times on the track that are better than I could do five or ten years ago. And, more important, it's joyful. I don't end a run in pain. Danny has a program that can truly revolutionize running."
          —Jerry Fletcher, Ed.D., age 61, Corte Madera, California

---

Also by Danny Dreyer and Katherine Dreyer

CHIWALKING: FITNESS WALKING FOR
LIFELONG HEALTH AND ENERGY

ChiRunning

A Revolutionary Approach to
Effortless, Injury-Free Running

Danny Dreyer
and Katherine Dreyer

A Fireside Book
Published by Simon & Schuster
New York London Toronto Sydney

This book is dedicated
to all our Teachers . . . you know who you are.

FIRESIDE
A Division of Simon & Schuster, Inc.
1230 Avenue of the Americas
New York, NY 10020

This Fireside trade paperback edition May 2009

FIRESIDE and colophon are registered trademarks of Simon & Schuster, Inc.

ChiRunning and ChiWalking are registered trademarks of ChiLiving, Inc.

For information about special discounts for bulk purchases,
please contact Simon & Schuster Special Sales at 1-866-506-1949 or
business@simonandschuster.com.

The Simon & Schuster Speakers Bureau can bring authors to your live event.
For more information or to book an event contact the Simon & Schuster Speakers Bureau
at 1-866-248-3049 or visit our website at www.simonspeakers.com.

Manufactured in the United States of America

10

Library of Congress Cataloging-in-Publication Data
Dreyer, Danny.
ChiRunning : a revolutionary approach to effortless, injury-free
running / Danny and Katherine Dreyer.
p.   cm.—(A Fireside book)
Originally published: c2004.
Includes bibliographical references and index.
1. Running—Training. 2. Tai chi. 3. Sports injuries—Prevention.
I. Dreyer, Katherine. II. Title. III. Title: Chi running.
GV1061.5.D74   2009
613.7'172—dc22   2009003793

ISBN-13: 978-1-4165-4944-4
ISBN-10:   1-4165-4944-7

Contents

Foreword
by Mark Cucuzzella, M.D.

I have been a runner since age 13 and ran competitively in college. My interest in medicine was sparked after experiencing our team physician try some very innovative, though unorthodox, approaches to treating running injuries. He was the first to have people run in the pool, and he built orthotics in his toaster oven. It seemed to him that there must be better ways to treat running injuries, so he blazed his own path. Oft-injured Mary Decker Slaney (former Olympian) was one of his patients to have a running rebirth by his methods. Runners now train in water, not just for injury rehab, but for low-impact supplemental training. And now, twenty years after my college racing, I am reviving the passion I felt at that time by witnessing how ChiRunning is giving many, including myself, a running rebirth.

We live in a sports medicine world where running injuries are still treated with rest, ice, stabilizing shoes, stretching, strengthening, and various rehab devices. But, despite all this *care*, runners are still getting injured at the same high rates. Many become former runners, not by choice, but out of suggestions from health practitioners selling them symptomatic relief instead of looking directly for the underlying causes of running injuries. Often the only solution offered is to stop running altogether. ChiRunning not only addresses the causes and cures of most running injuries, it teaches us a way to avoid them before they happen by changing how we run. This is the type of preventive medicine we all need to be moving toward.

I've been through my fair share of injury/recovery cycles too. In my younger years I had severe pain in both feet, subsequently requiring foot surgery in 2000 for severe arthritis. I could not dorsiflex (bend up) either great toe joints due to the degenerative changes. I thought my running days were over . . . as this was the orthopedic response to my injury. Perhaps take up another activity? No way. None were as convenient and relaxing as running.

Then in December 2005 I read an article in the Sunday *Washington Post* on ChiRunning. The short article was intriguing and led me to buy the book. After the first read and a little practice, I discovered what I had been missing in trying to find a way to run injury-free. Many of the cues were right in line with my other love, cross-country skiing. This was a method I could visualize completely.

Here was a succession of results *after* learning ChiRunning (*and the year I turned 40*).

- 2006 Boston Marathon (April)—53rd overall—2:31.45
- 2006 Ottawa Marathon (May)—8th overall—2:32.05
- 2006 Air Force Marathon (September)—1st overall—2:31.47
- 2006 Marine Corps Marathon (October)—11th overall, 1st Master—2:32.45

I ran four marathons (all 2:31–2:32) within six months, all feeling comfortable and with almost no recovery needed. There definitely was something to this technique, as I could not do this even in my younger years.

The beauty of focusing on form is that we can all continue to improve, sometimes in small steps but often in leaps. None of us has "perfect" running form, but I have seen and heard many stories from runners of all levels who practice the ChiRunning technique with astounding results.

I had the privilege of attending the four-day ChiRunning Instructor Course in October 2008. This immersion course accelerated my learning, and 2008 was one of the most successful fall running seasons in my life. But more important, I've learned how to better help others.

This method has given me running longevity, made it easier and painless, and has given me the confidence that I can run forever . . . into the retirement home. The ChiRunning methods are applied physics and biomechanics that any runner can apply to their benefit. "No pain, no gain" is now a thing of the past. "No pain, thank you." It's the ChiRunning way.

Mark Cucuzzella, M.D.,
FAAFP
Associate Professor of
Family Medicine, West
Virginia University
Lt. Col. U.S. Air Force
Reserves

Introduction to the New Edition

It has been five years since we wrote the first edition of *ChiRunning*. Since then almost two hundred thousand copies of the book have been sold in North America, and it has been translated into five languages and published in even more countries.

More important, it has helped hundreds of thousands of runners overcome injury and pain and find ease and joy in running once again. Beginning runners who had given up the struggle to try to run have discovered that running is possible for them. Success and excitement have replaced defeat and humiliation. Older runners who thought they had to quit found that they can continue to run. Successful athletes have found new speed and ease. Triathletes who have discovered ChiRunning don't dread the last leg of their event anymore. Countless physicians, chiropractors, physical therapists, and coaches have endorsed it and recommend ChiRunning to their clients.

We now have more than a hundred Certified ChiRunning Instructors, and their workshops are being taught all over the United States and in many other countries. You can find one near you at our website, www.chirunning.com.

Nothing has brought us more satisfaction than the letters we get from people. Publishing them would be an entire book in itself. You can read the most recent ones on our website. We are filled with gratitude to all of you who have helped make ChiRunning become a true revolution in the way people run. Here is a recent note—one of my favorites:

> Two and a half years now, ChiRunning. I have changed as a runner. Lately getting deeper into the feel of relaxation and the flow of Chi. I seem to have come a kind of full circle as I find that a single focus on the grounding stance as I run, one of your first lessons in your book, with the foot coming down one-third on the outside ball, one-third on the inside, and the other third on the heel, each foot feeling equal to the other in pressure and duration of ground contact, seems to align my posture, straighten my feet, set up the perfect lean, and is a very pleasing meditation on the quiet music my feet make on the Earth.
>
> —Joe Miller

This feels like poetry to me and captures the essence of ChiRunning. In December 2007 we did a survey with West Virginia University and Dr. Mark Cucuzella, a family practitioner (and 2:35 marathoner). We sent the survey to twenty-five thousand ChiRunning customers, and more than twenty-five hundred responded. Here are some of the results:

- 95% said their ease of running has improved
- 91% feel ChiRunning has played a role in preventing running injuries
- 90% said they were probably or definitely able to change their running mechanics with ChiRunning
- 61% said they were a heel-striker before practicing Chi-

Running, and 71% said they were a midfoot striker after practicing ChiRunning

- 60% said they were able to make noticeable corrections in less than a month, 31% said immediately
- 54% had an injury, and 88% with an injury said ChiRunning probably or definitely helped them recover
- 45% said their perceived exertion/discomfort before ChiRunning was very hard or hard, and less than 5% said their perceived exertion/discomfort was hard or very hard after practicing ChiRunning
- 69% felt their speed improved with ChiRunning
- Number of missed running days due to injury dropped dramatically: 40% had missed more than ten days prior to ChiRunning, while after ChiRunning that number dropped to less than 12%. Prior to ChiRunning 31% had no missed days, while after ChiRunning 61% had no missed days due to injury
- 91% said they would recommend ChiRunning to other runners

Further biomechanical studies of the ChiRunning technique are in the pipeline.

From the survey we also got a lot of information on how to help our clients learn this technique, and we've included all of this new information in this edition.

SETTING UP THE CONDITIONS FOR ENERGY TO FLOW

ChiRunning is all about setting up conditions that make running, easier, more efficient, and injury-free. We have discovered that in every aspect of our work, our teaching, and our own lives, creating the conditions for energy to flow is at the core of all our endeavors. If you set up the right conditions, then the rest follows easily. In ChiRunning, the primary setup is with your posture. When your posture is aligned, chi can flow up and down your spine and into your whole body. In my classes, if I set up the conditions for my clients to be at ease, then their learning process flows much more easily. We have been setting up the conditions for writing this new edition—getting feedback from our Certified Instructors and clients, going through all our notes from over the years, setting aside the best part of the day for the writing—and it is flowing from Katherine and me with an ease and enjoyment that has been delightful.

In this edition you'll be reading more about setting up the conditions to take your running to the next level of ease and enjoyment.

WHAT'S NEW IN THE NEW EDITION

The most important development that has occurred has been how we teach the ChiRunning technique. In every class and workshop I experiment to see how to get this information across in the clearest, easiest way possible. It is an ever-evolving process, just as learning and practicing this technique is an ongoing practice. In this new edition we are distilling all the information we have gleaned in teaching the method in our instructor courses and to thousands of clients over the past five years. Chapter 4, "Form Focuses," has been almost entirely rewritten to follow how I now teach a class and to explain exactly how to incorporate the Form Focuses into your running in the most efficient and easy-to-learn way, including ten lessons to get you started (Chapter 5).

One of the most significant developments since the original writing of this book has been the development of ChiWalking. I now teach ChiWalking as a part of every running class. We have found that everyone learns ChiRunning with greater ease when they are first introduced to ChiWalking. As we developed ChiWalking and wrote the ChiWalking book, *ChiWalking: Fitness Walking for Lifelong Health and Energy*, one of the key components of injury-free running emerged more fully: pelvic rotation.

Now, this may sound somewhat absurd. How can one concept, something so clinical and sterile-sounding (or maybe sexual), be so crucial to your running? The fact is that the stability and rotation of your pelvis around your centerline are probably two of the key factors in reducing injury, gaining core strength, and finding fluidity and speed in your stride. We expanded the explanation of pelvic rotation in this edition because we felt it was not given enough focus in the original edition. In the past five years we have discovered its incredible power. And, as we've mentioned, the pelvic rotation is most easily learned while walking.

Chapter 7, "Hills, Trails, and Treadmills" has all been updated and expanded upon, as has Chapter 9, "Troubleshooting: Injury Prevention and Recovery," where we present the ChiRunning solution to the most common running injuries.

THE MIDFOOT STRIKE

There is a rising consciousness in the running community about the midfoot strike. We have been teaching the midfoot strike to runners since 1999, but we did not emphasize it as a midfoot strike. In this edition the why and how of the midfoot strike are explained more fully.

THE PROCESS OF DISCOVERY: THE SUBTLETIES OF CHIRUNNING

What we have also learned is that although the ChiRunning technique is revolutionary as a concept, the learning of it should not be a revolution to your body but an evolution—that is, more a process of discovery than just following a set of rules. Leaning is a key concept of ChiRunning. However, the lean is very slight and each individual must find his or her own sweet spot. We teach you how to lean correctly, but it is part of *your* process to discover how it best works for you. Too much of a lean can cause your calves to clench up in pain. With the right amount of lean you can really begin to feel the potential effortlessness of running well.

The pelvic tilt (yes, more about the pelvis) is also a subtle movement. Many people don't think much about their pelvis, much less whether it is tilting or not. However, discovering the sweet spot of your pelvic tilt by Body Sensing (Chapter 3) is a self-discovery that will add years to your running, improve your overall posture, keep your hips and lower back healthy, stave off hip replacements and iliotibial band syndrome, and do a host of other good deeds for your body. Too much of a pelvic tilt may cause a lower-back ache. The pelvic tilt is a subtle movement and we'll give you all the information we can in this book, on the DVD, and in workshops, but ultimately it is up to you to discover your own perfect pelvic tilt.

Gradual Progress: A Practice and a Process

We get lots of letters from clients telling us that after reading just a few chapters of the book they are running faster than ever, beating their previous personal records and feeling less effort. That is wonderful. However we always ask those folks to follow the theme of Gradual Progress and come back to us in six months or a year and let us know how it's going. We ask them to take their time, integrate the changes slowly and carefully, check in with their bodies regularly, and discover over time what really works best for them. Just a few of the ChiRunning practices can have a huge positive effect on your running, but the deep work of integration means practicing these techniques over time.

We now have clients who have been using this method since 1999, when I first began to teach the technique in the San Francisco Bay area. I am pleased to say we get lots of letters from them too, telling us how their running is still injury-free and better than ever from years of instilling these practices into their lives and into their walking and into their running. Those are the letters we cherish the most, as the practices are time-tested.

Katherine and I have a deep sense of joy that we have helped lots of people with their running. We know that having a safe and solid running program can make a huge difference in the quality of your life. There is nothing like a run to make you feel alive, vibrant, and at peace. ChiRunning helps you come to that wonderful place of inner strength and certainty without the worry of hurting your body.

We hope you enjoy this new edition as much as we've enjoyed writing it. And we send our deep gratitude to all of you who have spread the word by sharing ChiRunning with friends and family.

Running Lessons from a T'ai Chi Master

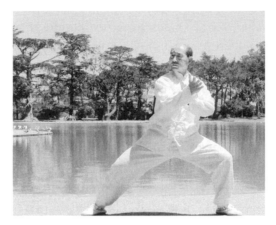

Master George Xu

Not long ago, I was running past a grade school. It was a warm late spring day, and the kids were out on recess. They were busy playing tag, chasing balls, and just doing what kids do best, running around. I stopped to take a swig of water from my bottle, and as I watched the flurry of little legs, I was reminded once again why I love to watch kids run. Every one of them had perfect running form: a nice lean, a great stride opening up behind them, heels high in the air, relaxed arm swing and shoulders. They had it all!

RUN LIKE A CHILD

One of my biggest desires as a coach is to help adults learn to run the way they did as kids. It's such a natural movement when kids do it. It looks so effortless and joyful. Many books about running tell you to

just go out and run like you did as a kid. There's only one problem
with that suggestion: you don't have the same body today that you did
back then. If you do, I'd like you to be my teacher.

So why don't adults run like kids, with that same ease and joyful-
ness? After running for thirty years and working with thousands of
runners, I'd have to say that the two biggest factors are stress and tension. I can speak for myself, and maybe you can relate. Since I left the
sixth grade, I have put my body through a wide range of physical and
emotional stresses, such as tightening my shoulders when I'm wor-
ried, slouching all day at my desk, holding tension in my neck while
driving—the list is endless. Individually, these might not sound like a
big deal, but when you add them all up over a lifetime, they have a
major cumulative effect on how you move. I've also done a few radical
things that have taken a bit more of a toll on my body, like skiing off
cliffs and doing face plants while skateboarding. As Caroline Myss,
author of *Anatomy of the Spirit*, would say, "Your biography becomes
your biology." With all of this abuse stored in my body, I'd be hard
pressed to run the way I did as a kid. The good news is that for anyone
with a little patience and perseverance, it is possible to get back to
that state.

There are more than 24 million runners in the United States alone.
But get this. It is estimated that 65% of all runners incur at least one
injury a year that interrupts their training. That means that 15.6 million people will get injured this year from running. No wonder people
have a love/hate relationship with running. It's one of the most ac-
cessible and inexpensive ways to stay in shape, yet it poses a danger
that is cautioned about in articles, books, and doctors' offices every-
where. Most people treat injury as part of the sport and learn to accept that it will happen sooner or later: "I'll deal with it when it
happens." It's the same line I get when I ask people in the San Francisco Bay area if they worry about earthquakes.

The conclusion I've come to after teaching countless runners is
that *running does not hurt your body*. Let me repeat that—and you
can read my lips—*running does not hurt your body*. It's the *way* you
run that does the damage and causes pain.

When Adriane, 42, came to me, she was caught in a back-and-forth cycle of training hard to get into good condition, then getting injured and having to lay off for a couple of weeks, and finally starting all over again. She thought it was the right thing to constantly train fast and strength-train to improve her times in the marathon. But she was not making any forward progress because of the nagging injuries and her own internal pressure to keep increasing her weekly race-training schedule. With the ChiRunning technique, she learned how to relax while running and, more important, in the other areas of her life. She realized that she was not only a driven runner, she was a driven person. Without all the tension in her body, she stopped injuring herself while running, and her training took on a new level of consistency.

Jerry, a 59-year-old runner, was just about to give up running when he came to his first ChiRunning class. He had been a runner for forty years, and after having knee surgery, he had begun to feel the same old aches and pains creeping into his runs that had prompted the surgery. He was afraid that if he continued running, he would ruin his knees and live in pain for the rest of his life. It has now been two years since his first class, and he is running regularly—including an hour and a half on steep trails once a week—and looking forward to many more years of pleasurable running.

Carmen, 35, was a beginning runner and insecure about her ability to do anything well physically. After taking a series of three ChiRunning classes, she happened to call as my wife, Katherine, and I were reviewing her class on video. Katherine remarked on how good Carmen looked in the film and asked her how she liked the class. "Oh, it simply changed my life" was the reply. "For the first time in my life, I feel like I can be good at a sport."

From beginners to competitors to the forty-plus crowd who are afraid of injuring themselves as they get older, ChiRunning is meeting the needs of runners with an approach that builds a healthy body instead of breaking it down from misuse or overuse.

ChiRunning Versus Power Running

The current paradigm of running form and injury prevention is founded in muscle strength. It is basically built around three principles: (1) if you want to run faster, you need to build stronger leg muscles; (2) if you want to run longer, you need to build stronger leg muscles; (3) if you want to avoid or recover from injuries, you need to build stronger leg muscles. Do you see a theme developing here? It's all dependent on muscles to get the job done, and the leg muscles are given the bulk of the responsibility to make it all happen. That's a lot of responsibility and, according to T'ai Chi principles, a very unbalanced way to move your body. The problem with strength training is that it doesn't get to the root of the most common cause of injury: poor running form. Most runners want to run either longer or faster at some point in their running career, but without good running form, added distance will only lengthen the time you are running improperly and increase your odds of getting hurt. If you try to add speed with improper running form, you are magnifying the poor biomechanical habits that could cause injury. So the best place to build a good foundation is in getting your running motion smooth, relaxed, and efficient. Then you can add distance or speed without risking injury.

This book presents an alternative to what we call power running. ChiRunning is based on the centuries-old principle from T'ai Chi that states, *Less is more*. Getting back to that childhood way of running doesn't come from building bigger muscles; it comes from relaxing muscles, opening tight joints, and using gravity to do the work instead of pushing and forcing your body to move in ways that can do it harm. Most runners, especially those over 35, will tell you that running can keep you in good shape but it's hard on your body. I developed ChiRunning because I really didn't believe that pounding and injury should be a part of running. I just didn't buy it.

THE DISCOVERY OF CHIRUNNING

I've never considered myself a great runner. I liked to run as a kid, but I shied away from it in high school because, to tell you the truth, I was intimidated by the caliber of our track team members, most of whom could run a hundred-yard dash in under ten seconds and a quarter mile in under a minute. In an inner-city high school with 2,600 students, the coaches could basically pick from the cream of the crop, and I hardly considered myself even potential cream. So I joined the ski club and partied instead. In fact, I signed up to take gymnastics, because every Wednesday the gym classes had to run around a nearby lake, and I couldn't imagine making myself run for twelve minutes without stopping.

Don't get me wrong. I've always loved sports, and I love to learn new things with my body. Whenever I wanted to take on a new sport, I would apply another love of mine—figuring out how things work. As far back as I can remember, I've always had questions running through my mind, like "Why does a clock tick?" or "What kind of machine wraps a stick of butter?" As a kid, I loved taking things apart to see what made them do what they did, and then I'd try to put them back together again. Although I had a lifetime average of about 75% on the reassembly, I always figured out how they worked.

This is what I did with skiing, rock climbing, and sailing. I broke each sport down into its elemental parts, which would then give me a physical understanding of how to put it all together into a unified movement. As I found myself improving, I would get more excited and consequentially focus even more. My learning was driven by my passion, so my hours spent practicing would fly by. I loved learning new body skills.

In my early twenties, when I took up running, I approached it in much the same way. I began running regularly in 1971, when I got drafted into the army. Running around the army base at an easy pace was very relaxing for my body and helped to settle my mind. This was the first time I had used a sport for more than physical fitness: I wasn't into being in the army, so I used running to escape the barracks and explore. After doing an eighteen-week stint with Uncle Sam, I was graciously given an honorable discharge, but not before discovering a new favorite pastime.

When I was a young adult, my curiosity about how things worked extended into those unseen forces out of which the physical world springs forth. I was no longer satisfied with only understanding the *how*; I wanted to know *why* they worked. I always came away with a sense that there was more going on than I was seeing. For lack of a better term, I call it the invisible world, and my curiosity about it is still the driving force behind my approach to life. It eventually led me to the study of T'ai Chi and using chi in my running.

The same year I started running, I began my investigation of the invisible by practicing long hours of meditation with a teacher from India. The most important knowledge I gained was how to quiet my mind so I could listen to my body. As my meditation practice began to spill into my running, my running became more and more an exploration of my own physical nature and the energies powering it.

Fast-forward to 1991. Over a period of twenty years, my running and my exploration of the invisible had become increasingly intertwined. I began running longer and longer distances as a means of exploring the potential of my body, which is what led me to the sport of ultramarathon running (distances longer than 26.2 miles). In 1995 I ran my first race, a 50-miler in Boulder, Colorado. Since then I have completed forty ultramarathons, winning my age group in fourteen of them and placing in the top three in my age group in all but one. The distances I have raced are 50K (31 miles), 50 miles, 100K (62 miles), and 100 miles. In 2002 I ran my first marathon (the Big Sur International Marathon), winning my age group in a time of 3:04, which I was very pleased with, considering there's about a thousand feet of vertical gain on the course.

Now, I just have to say right here that the ChiRunning technique is *not* about running superlong distances. I have chosen ultradistance running as a way to learn about my body, but I don't necessarily recommend it for everyone. If you are so inclined, ChiRunning certainly makes distance running more enjoyable, but even more important, it represents a way to move your body by using mental focus and relaxation instead of muscle power. In this book you will learn about the principle of "form, distance, and speed," which means that you start by building a foundation of correct running form. As your foundation gets stronger, your body will be able to handle more distance. Then speed becomes a by-product of good technique practiced over increased distance, not something dependent on the size and strength of your muscles. Ultimately, you're not working to build distance and speed, you're working to build *presence*, and that can happen at any distance or speed.

When I first started running ultras, they were hard work. Along the way I had bouts with aches and pains, which I tried to approach with a positive attitude, telling myself, "If you can get this right, you might not have this pain again." At one point in my training, I had a knee pain that would start about 20 miles into my long run. But I never blamed the running for injuring my body. Instead, I took full responsibility by always trying to figure out how my form was causing my knees to hurt. I assumed that it was a matter of making the right correction, and I let that premise guide me in my trial-and-error research.

T'AI CHI LESSONS

In 1997 my eyes were opened to a whole new realm when I met Zhu Xilin, a T'ai Chi master from China who introduced me to the concept of moving from one's center and letting the arms and legs follow. His way of moving his body looked both effortless and powerful. Needless to say, adapting this idea to my running was a huge draw for me.

T'ai Chi owes its origins to the study of animal movements. According to the Chinese, chi (pronounced "chee") is the energy force that animates all things. It runs through a system of meridians that distribute this energy to all parts of your body. By practicing mental focus and relaxation, one can learn to sense and direct this subtle energy through the system of movements and exercises known as T'ai Chi. This concept is downplayed by Western medicine because chi cannot be detected with measuring instruments and cannot be supported by the scientific method. The interesting part about chi is that it will move through your body whether you believe in it or not, because if it weren't running through you, you'd be dead. Fair enough?

The current trend in sports training toward using one's core muscles is just starting to scratch the surface of knowledge the Chinese have been developing for more than two thousand years. One of the things T'ai Chi teaches us is to direct movement from points along our spine; thus it can originate from the centerline of your body and not from the periphery. Observation of Nature teaches us that the strength of a tree lies in its trunk, not in the branches and leaves.

Why should the human body be any different? Why do you think the area of your body that houses all your vital organs is called your trunk? Are we nodding yet?

Look at the movement of a cheetah, the fastest land animal on earth. It doesn't have big strong legs like a tiger. It has skinny legs like a greyhound. So how does it go so fast? The secret lies in its spine, which is where most of its chi is contained. When a cheetah runs, you can see that its source of power comes from the spine and not the legs.

For your legs to be powered by the chi coming through the spine, they need to be very relaxed. Master Zhu would constantly tell me to keep my spine straight but relax the rest of my body and let the chi flow through "like water through a pipe." A major lightbulb went on in my head when it occurred to me that this idea could be applied to running.

I started to grasp the idea of moving my body from its center and letting my legs be pulled along for the ride. But relaxing my arms and legs while running only uncovered the next problem in the chain— the need to relax my shoulders and hips. Once I became adept at relaxing, I could feel how much power my spine had when it wasn't met with any resistance from the rest of my body. That was when I began to experience a new level of smoothness and ease, often feeling as if I were skimming along on a conveyor belt. As I worked on technique, my sense of running more smoothly and efficiently gradually began to replace that old feeling of working hard to run. My breathing became less labored, my muscles were not getting sore, and many times I would feel better at the end of a run than I did when I started. I could go out for a thirty-mile run and come back without any major discomfort: an exhilarating realization. "Post-run recovery" began to take on a whole new meaning—hours instead of days, and sometimes no time at all. This is when I realized that I was on to something *very* cool. Since my discovery in 1998, I have not had a running injury of any kind (knock on wood), despite a heavy teaching, training, and racing schedule.

In 1999 I moved from Boulder to San Francisco, feeling a great sense of loss at having to leave Master Zhu. When I first arrived, I ran through Golden Gate Park, looking for a new T'ai Chi teacher. Each day I'd see many small groups practicing their moves, and there would be Master Xu, who always had only one student. He would be manually moving his subject into various postures, like an artist shaping a clay figure. He was totally attentive to his student in a way that I never witnessed in any of the other teachers. After seeing him numerous times at the same spot, I decided to ask him if he would be my teacher. I introduced myself and said, "I don't care if I ever learn T'ai Chi, but I want to learn how to apply what *you* do to my running." His face lit up. "I've always had a theory," he said, "that one could take all the principles of T'ai Chi and use them in any sport. Come back in three months."

That was it. He never gave me his name or phone number. Just "Come back in three months." What could I say? So, after ninety days of waiting, I went back and found him in the same spot where I left him. I reminded him who I was, to which he responded, "Okay, start tomorrow." I fully expected him to end his sentence with "grasshopper." As it turns out, George Xu is an internationally known T'ai Chi master who leads seminars all over the world and has produced an extensive collection of videotapes documenting many Chinese masters of almost every martial art in China. Since that day, Master Xu (pronounced "shoe") has had a huge impact on the further development of what I have come to call ChiRunning. He has not only confirmed and clarified all that I'd discovered prior to meeting him, he has helped me to synthesize the themes of T'ai Chi with what I've learned about running.

I've always loved to watch people run. It's wonderful to see how many different types of bodies there are and how many different ways they run. But if you want to see what's really going on with a runner, watch her face. If you watch children run, they're generally all smiles. But what I see more often than not in adults is an expression that ranges somewhere between discomfort and terror. Lots of folks leave me with the impression that they're not enjoying themselves. No wonder running has a bad rap. What happened to all those smiles?

We need to reeducate ourselves to move in the ways we were designed to move. Most people are never taught how to run. It's one of those things we all take for granted because everyone runs soon after learning to walk. Go to any fitness center, gym, or continuing-education catalog, and you'll find classes in every sport on the planet *except* running. This was a big part of what convinced me to become a full-time coach and running instructor. As I brought more of the inner focuses of T'ai Chi into my running classes, the students began to see immediate and dramatic changes in their performance and outlook. Since introducing the ChiRunning technique to the general public, I've seen many of those smiles reappear.

Through my T'ai Chi teachers, I have learned that losing the beautiful ease of movement we had as children is part of the process of maturing as a human being. Children move naturally but not consciously. It is our job, as adults, to learn how to move consciously through life with that same flow and beauty. It is through conscious action and understanding that we can become masters of our bodies and ourselves. The ChiRunning technique is the vehicle that will allow you to experience once again what it's like to run with a sense of power and connection in your body.

I still don't consider myself an exceptional runner. When I run, I rely almost entirely on inner focuses and technique rather than on talent or physical strength. Ultimately, ChiRunning is not about being an accomplished runner; it's about what you come away with. It's learning how to listen to your body and adjust appropriately to improve your form and enhance your performance. It's learning how to sense your body, your actions, and the results of your actions; how to learn from what you do and what you feel. It's learning how to use running as a vehicle to discover yourself on many levels.

If you would like to improve your running form, have fewer injuries, develop your own training program, and be able to run into your old age, then this book is for you.

If you would like to increase your overall health and well-being, this book is for you too.

If you would like to learn to be more centered and have more of a mindful approach to your running and your life, this book is also for you. ChiRunning is not so much about the running as it is about the chi. It's about having a focused and energetic relationship with your body. It means learning how to be your own best friend, teacher, and guide—how to be mindful, quiet, and energetic all at the same time. Sound great? It is.

How to Use This Book

I'd like to take a minute here and clue you in on what to expect in the coming chapters. As a fair warning, I do not get into explaining the technique of ChiRunning until Chapter 4. So if it feels like I'm taking forever to get to the good stuff, there's a reason. Not only does this book tell you how to be a better runner, it also offers you the opportunity to develop qualities from running that you can use in the rest of your life. This approach to running is best understood when you can see the background and logic supporting it. The first three chapters are dedicated to laying out the philosophical foundation, so when I give you the specifics of the technique, they will all make sense.

Chapter 1 compares the present paradigm of running, power running, to ChiRunning, the proverbial new kid on the block. Chapter 2 introduces you to the three principles, or natural laws, upon which T'ai Chi and ChiRunning are based. When your movements are in sync with the laws of Nature, you have one of the best support systems around, to put it mildly. And Chapter 3 will explain to you the "inner" skills of ChiRunning, which I call Chi-Skills. Learning these four mind/body skills will change your running into an entirely new activity.

Chapter 4 introduces you to the ChiRunning focuses, which are the specific physical and mental methods used to run more smoothly, efficiently, and injury-free. Chapter 5 gives you ten lessons that show you how to take the Form Focuses of Chapter 4 and bring them into your running in a time-tested, sequential way.

Chapters 6–11 teach you how to bring the ChiRunning technique into your running program, including program development, peak performance training, advanced focuses, and diet. Chapter 12 then tells you how to bring the ChiRunning principles into your everyday life.

I would suggest reading the book straight through once. Then go back and reread portions that are not clear to you. My favorite trick with a manual is to mark all of my favorite sections with a tab, labeled for easy reference. If you want something more permanent and reliable, go to your local office-supply store, buy some stick-on plastic tabs, and go crazy. I'd mark all the exercises, drills, focuses, and tips so you can access the information easily if you're on your way out the door for a run. Believe me, you will use this book more often if you have a system in which the information is at your fingertips. You'll find the ChiRunning DVD, online training programs, support from ChiRunning Certified Instructors, and a host of other training tools on our website, ChiRunning.com.

I've found that the body and mind learn best through repetition. For this reason, I recommend that you reread this book several times, then at least once a year, to keep your mind and body refreshed with the process and terminology. Take your time, and you'll learn more, faster.

Learning the basic ChiRunning technique can take anywhere from one to six months for the average runner, but the greater knowledge gained from the approach will be something that, when practiced regularly, will influence your thoughts and actions for the rest of your life.

CHAPTER ONE

ChiRunning: A Revolution in Running

A good runner leaves no footprints. —LAO TZU

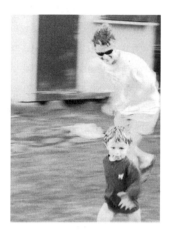

As Emily ran past our group at the track, we all remarked at what beautiful running form she had. She seemed to float across the ground so effortlessly that you could hardly hear her feet touch down. The moment seemed almost otherworldly, and she became the role model for everyone in the class because of her beautiful running form.

Emily is a 3-year-old whose parents were taking a ChiRunning class at the track that day.

Children run naturally. When they want to catch their friends in a game of tag, all they do is focus on who's It and their body just follows along. They're not thinking about running. They're enjoying the game of tag and having so much fun that there is very little actual work going on when they're running. And since very little effort is involved in their movement, there is little chance for injury. There isn't

13

any pounding in their joints or any tension in their muscles that could be the hot spots for pain to reside. How *could* there be when their movement is based on fun and play?

Sarah Hughes, upon winning the gold medal in women's figure skating at the 2002 Olympics, said, "I wasn't thinking of a gold medal, I went out to have fun and a great time. . . . All I wanted to do was skate my best." It was easy to see how much fun she was having. Her sense of freedom and joy allowed the energy in her body to fill the arena, infectiously sparking the audience. On the other hand, Michelle Kwan, five-time world champion, was caught by the camera just as she was about to go on the ice. The anxiety in her face displayed the pressure she was under to produce a gold medal for her country. She looked anything but relaxed and playful. My heart went out to her. The tension that she was carrying prevented her best energy from moving through her body, resulting in a performance below what she was capable of and landing her the bronze medal.

I would venture to say that most of us could run pretty easily back when we were in grade school and not feeling pressured to perform. But we have since lost that wonderful sense of ease. Like Michelle, we often have performance anxiety that makes us uptight and blocks us from feeling ourselves and doing our best. In order to regain this ease and joy, we need to consciously teach our bodies how to relax and move so that running can feel as effortless as it once did.

A great way for me to learn to relax has been my study of what I call the perceived rate of exertion (PRE). Your PRE is the amount of exertion you sense yourself to be doing. Let's say that Joan is an average runner in decent shape. She goes out for her morning run and puts in a few miles at a 9:00 minutes-per-mile pace. She's been doing it for weeks and she has a distinct physical sensation of what that particular pace feels like. To her it feels like a nice, comfortable, easy pace. Then she goes to a party that evening and dances to some great rock and roll after having a couple of beers. The next morning she drags herself out of bed to run with her next-door neighbor who also likes to run at a 9:00 pace. As they get into their run she asks him how fast they're going, because it feels like a bit much. He tells her that they're exactly on pace—9:00 on the button. Meanwhile, she's feeling like she's trying to hustle to catch a crosstown bus. Her legs are tired, she's breathing like a freight train, and she's not sure how much longer she can keep it up. Her PRE feels *way* higher than it was yesterday, but they're running the exact same pace.

Your PRE is what you *feel* like you're doing regardless of what you are *actually* doing. The emphasis of ChiRunning is to set yourself up so that there are no blocks and your energy can freely flow through your body. This is accomplished by (1) maintaining good posture, (2) keeping your joints open and loose, and (3) making sure that your muscles are relaxed and not holding any tension as you run. If you're practicing these, your PRE will feel lower than it normally does, at whatever speed you're running. As your running form becomes increasingly efficient you will run faster and/or longer with *less* perceived effort. There's no reason why getting into great shape needs to hurt or feel strenuous. And, there's no reason on earth why it can't be fun. As your ability to run well increases, so will your sense of joy. And likewise, as your joy increases, so does your ability to run well.

The ChiRunning technique will completely alter the way you approach running because it combines relaxation with biomechanically correct running form. This book is designed to train your mind to direct and monitor your movements so that your body doesn't have to work as hard. One of my favorite quotes from Master Xu reflects this perfectly: *"The body wears out . . . the mind lasts forever."*

Here's a sample exercise that will give you a sense of PRE. It will help you feel the difference between using lots of leg muscles to move your legs (hard work/higher PRE) and using your core muscles to do the same (easy work/lower PRE).

- Set this book down and stand up straight and tall.
- Walk in place for 10 seconds, picking up your feet.
- After walking in place for 10 seconds, bend over at the waist— like you're bowing—and walk in place for another 10 seconds.
- Now straighten your body to the vertical position and keep walking in place for a few seconds.

How did it feel to "walk" bent over? How did it feel when you straightened up your body? Was it any easier? If you sense in your body that standing tall while picking up your feet is the easier way to go, it's because it is.

Here's what's happening. When you're standing tall and upright, your psoas (pronounced "so as") muscles are stretched and act somewhat like a rubber band to lift your leg when you walk in place. Those are two of the strongest core muscles in your body, working to lift the weight of your feet, which means that there's a *large* muscle group doing a *tiny* job. When you bend over at the waist, your psoas is disengaged and you have to lift the weight of your leg with your quadriceps, which is more work.

This exercise is intended to give you a sense of how much harder your legs have to work if you're bent over at the waist, and not holding your posture in a straight line. In Chapter 4, I will talk about how to take your nice straight posture and tilt it forward while running, which will lower your PRE even more.

Before I get into telling you more about how running is going to be easier for you, let's talk about why you would want to run at all.

THE BENEFITS OF RUNNING

I might sound like a fanatic, but I love running. It's like having an old friend that is always there when you need a lift in spirits. Once I get myself out the door the world opens, no matter how hemmed in or bummed out I might be feeling. I can call up a friend to come along and explore a new trail or spend a morning cruising canyons and watching waterfalls. Running gets you outside, and if you run all year long, it does a wonderful job of keeping you in touch with the changes of the seasons.

Oh, and you know what else happens while I'm out there having the time of my life? My heart gets stronger, my bone density increases, I burn a ton of calories, and my aerobic capacity improves. Not bad for a day of play.

It's inexpensive and requires minimal gear. You can run almost anytime and anywhere. There is nothing like a good run to clear your mind and put life's problems into a better perspective. When you travel to a new city it's a great way to learn the lay of the land and get an intimate feel for your new surroundings. And there is no better way to cleanse your body of overindulgences.

You can also develop qualities from running that can be transferred into the rest of your life, including perseverance, consistency, and willpower. Maintaining a solid running program can teach you how to set goals and work toward them, how to develop a strategic action plan, or how to use setbacks as lessons to be learned. In fact, there is almost no situation in your life that cannot be approached and handled from what you learn about yourself through running. Running can truly be a study of life itself.

WHY PEOPLE GET INJURED

For all the good that can be gained from running, it is also fraught with many potential dangers to your body. It can damage your knees, shins, hips, and back. It can take its toll on your feet, and it's even been said that it can damage your eyesight from all the jarring and pounding. People are led to believe that running inherently creates these types of injuries. That's a myth I would like to put to sleep.

The most common theory says that the primary cause of running injuries is overtraining. I also believe this to be a myth, although it is a factor, especially in results-oriented training. I believe the primary cause of injury is poor running form and poor biomechanics. Running is a natural movement. Having poor biomechanics means that you are moving your body in an unnatural way. This will lead to undue stress on muscles, joints, and ligaments which can then become vulnerable to injury. If you have poor running form, you can injure yourself at any distance. I've seen people get shin splints after half a mile. If there is an imperfection in your biomechanics, it will eventually show up as an ache or pain. You only need to run far enough and each of those little imperfections will eventually take their toll on your body. I guarantee it.

The upside is, if you improve your biomechanics and your running form, you greatly decrease your odds of getting injured at *any* distance or speed.

Paul, age 35, was an average runner who wanted to challenge himself by completing a marathon. The farthest he had ever gone was 6 miles because every time he ran, his shins would start hurting to the point where they hobbled him. He told me that they actually started hurting within the first mile of every run. He came to his first ChiRunning class in July with a goal of running the Honolulu Marathon in early December. With the help of the ChiRunning technique he was able to run all of his mileage upgrades while decreasing the pain level in his shins. After months of dedicating himself to practicing his new running form, he was able to run his *first* marathon in 3:37 without the debilitating pain of his shin splints. He told me later that he would not have thought it possible to complete a marathon before working on his form. Now he's thinking of trying to qualify for the Boston Marathon!

The current paradigm of running technique is, I believe, why there are so many injuries incurred by runners. We call it power running.

POWER RUNNING: NO PAIN, NO GAIN

No doubt about it, that macho catchphrase is still getting airtime, like it's some kind of badge of honor. It doesn't matter whether you're talking about running programs, international relations, or making a pie crust—there are better ways to approach almost any activity than by force.

Power running can best be explained by looking at it from two angles: technique and mind-set. Both the technique and mind-set of power running are reflected in the "no pain, no gain" attitude that pervades Western sports and thinking. Don't get me wrong. Power running does work, but it can be quite costly in terms of energy expenditure and injury rates. I just keep thinking about the more than 16 million runners who are getting injured *each year*, and I know that doesn't have to be the case.

THE POWER RUNNING METHOD

The predominant theme of power running is to develop leg strength and leg speed in order to run faster and farther. Power running emphasizes regular training to get your legs stronger, which will help you to run better. There are many exercise plans designed to build stronger calves, more powerful quads, and buns of steel so that you can become a better runner.

From a training standpoint, building and using more muscles is in itself hard work for the body and even more difficult for us folks over 40. Any increase in muscle usage requires that more time be spent on strength training and creates a greater propensity for injury. Additionally, more fuel is required to power these muscles, more metabolic waste (lactic acid) is produced, and subsequently more time is needed for recovery after running, especially after races or hard workouts. It makes me tired and achy just thinking about it.

I read about a comparative study done in Denmark that looked at the difference between Danish runners and Kenyan runners. Here's what they had to say, according to an article in the *Kampala Monitor*.

In all, it was discovered that Kalenjin (Kenyan) elite runners as well as untrained Kalenjin boys have a superior running economy compared to their Danish counterparts probably due to the fact that the Kalenjins have more slender legs and thus use relatively less energy when running.

They got part of it right. The Kenyans are using relatively less energy, but it's not because their legs are skinny. It's really the other way around. Their legs are slender *because* they have such excellent running economy. They're so efficient they don't need big leg muscles. Their calves are the size of my forearm and their quads are the size of my biceps . . . and I don't have big arms to begin with. The Kenyans are winning everything from 10Ks to marathons with those "slender legs." I'd say it's their technique that is winning races, a technique that shares many of the characteristics of ChiRunning, including their lean and foot strike. The Kenyans have a beautiful forward lean when they run, which does two things. It allows gravity to assist in pulling their body forward, and it allows them to land with a midfoot strike, avoiding the overuse of their calf muscles. They also have a strong core because of their forward lean and a full pelvic rotation, which is a central part of the ChiRunning form—you'll learn about it in Chapter 4.

From an injury standpoint, power running can be detrimental to runners because it does not address the real cause of most injuries, which is poor biomechanics. Instead it focuses almost entirely on building stronger muscles as a solution for recovering from or avoiding injures. It's true, strengthening muscles will buy you some time. But until you correct the real inefficiencies in your running technique, your running will require more work from your muscles and create more impact to your joints. And odds are you're going to get the same injury again.

For instance, if you have shin splints, you can take time off to heal them and then spend time strengthening the tibialis anterior (shin muscle) by walking on your heels. But if you're still using the same running form that created the shin splints, you run a pretty high risk of getting them again. With the ChiRunning technique, you won't be pushing off with your toes (one of the primary causes of shin splints) and you'll rarely use your shin muscles. Shin splints will become a nonissue and you won't have to build and maintain stronger muscles to compensate for your running form.

Almost everyone I see is power running (except the Kenyans, soccer players, and anyone under 8 years old), and for decades "vertical running" has been the approach to running used by every level of coach from middle school through college. But when I think of that statistic of running having a 65% yearly injury rate, I can't help thinking that there is something seriously wrong with the way we're approaching running. What is needed is a paradigm shift, away from the power running approach. ChiRunning represents that shift.

THE POWER RUNNING MIND-SET

The conventional mind-set of most power runners is "results oriented," which I feel is the primary cause of overtraining. People get ideas in their heads about how fast or far they should run that are not necessarily based on a reality in their body.

This is not only a setup for disappointment—it's a recipe for injury. Overtraining can be defined as training beyond the level at which your body is currently capable. That means that if you're a beginning runner and you pick up a training program that says you should be running 2 miles three days a week, you could be a candidate for over-training. What if you've never run a mile?

If you're driven to do more than you're capable of, you are usually driven by something *external* to yourself. It could be a desire triggered by an inspirational article in a running magazine, or an impulse you get from watching a great athlete on TV. Here are some of the faces of external motivators:

- Wanting to do better because of peer pressure
- Trying to match the speed of your running partners
- Wishing to be faster than you were last year
- Needing to prove your value to your parents
- Wanting to keep up with your significant other
- Trying to lose those last fifteen pounds before your wedding day
- Hoping to run a marathon by a certain age or date
- Trying to keep up with your dog

The list is endless. And in case you didn't notice, they're all products of a results-oriented mind-set.

There are plenty of external reasons to motivate you, but the motivators that really get things rolling and generate successes are the ones that come from *inside* you. Unfortunately, our Western culture is becoming increasingly shaped by the world of marketing, which has at its roots the mission to pull you off your center and outside yourself so that you'll buy whatever product or service is put before your eyes. Power running books and magazines promote the images that we are constantly bombarded with, like "bigger is better," "survival of the fittest," and everybody's favorite, "no pain, no gain." Just look at the cover of any current running or fitness magazine and you'll be hit with alluring catchphrases like "You too can have ripped abs!" or

"Have a hard body in six days!" Right . . . but what about those of us who are over 18?

The Chi in ChiRunning

I'm sure there are people you've seen in your life who have had the uncanny ability to perform at a skill level that seemed to be leagues beyond their nearest peer. They're the ones that can make a difficult activity look like child's play. Anyone who has that high level of connection to their body is doing it by directing their chi, whether or not they know it. It's a highly developed skill that might have come easily to them, but it's a skill nonetheless. There are a few people of this caliber that come to mind for me. One of my favorite people to watch was Barry Sanders, a running back for the Detroit Lions. He could weave his way to the goal line through a crowd of 300-pound defenders who were totally bent on his demise, and make it look like everyone was in slow motion but himself. He had the focus of a heat-seeking missile and the lightness of a cat. He could change directions quicker than one thought humanly possible, and I loved to watch how he could stay on his feet and keep his balance through what seemed like unearthly challenges. Even though he probably didn't think about using chi to make his way to the goal line, he was a master at moving his body with the focus and speed of his mind . . . very much a principle straight out of T'ai Chi.

Barry Sanders, Serena Williams, Yo-Yo Ma, Michael Phelps, Meryl Streep, Tiger Woods, Apolo Ohno—these are people who might make you say, "Wow . . . it's unbelievable what they can do with their body! How do they do that and make it look so damned easy?" From interviews that I've heard, my understanding of how they do it is that they don't *do* anything. They simply get themselves out of the way and allow something else to happen. Not everyone on this list is an athlete, but they're all highly skilled in their craft, to the point of making it an art form. Their high level of skill allows them to cross over into further realms of physical expression and movement, beyond where most of us are capable of going. They can go there because they no longer need to think about what they have to do in the midst of a challenge. When their mind moves, their body follows. If their focus moves, their chi goes with it, and everything that needs to happen takes place as it should without the interference of doubt, anxiety, tension, fears, or ego, which could dampen the actions of those less skilled in their craft.

Whenever I get to meet Master Xu for another lesson, he gives me example after example of how the power of chi is stronger than muscle. Over and over he tosses my body around like I'm a feather, without using any visible physical effort. His muscles don't tense up as he moves me. He's just moving his body as if I wasn't there, and if my body happens to be in the path of his arm, I get flattened. He never breaks a sweat or even breathes hard. All he says is, "I let chi do it." Then he says, "Just set up your body correctly and let the chi move through it. Let your mind do the work . . . let your body relax. Don't let muscles do it. Let chi do it."

Chi is also known as life-force energy. It generates movement in the physical world and is that which animates life. It is also the energy that is created by movement, so it is both the product and the tool. It is the life-giving energy that unites body, mind, and spirit, an invisible and nonmeasurable force that can be seen only by the effect that it has, like air, which can be seen only when it blows through the leaves of a tree or inflates a balloon.

I love to garden, but like any other gardener, I can't make the plants grow. The best I can do is to provide the optimal conditions for growth to happen. I can plant the seed in a place that gets good sunlight, add compost to condition the soil, and make sure that there's plenty of water to nourish the young seedling. Each of these steps helps to ensure that chi will infuse the seed with enough life force to sprout. Somewhere in a dessert, a seed can lie dormant for thousands of years in a clay pot at the bottom of an Indian ruin. But it won't sprout unless there is enough chi to get things moving. That's my job as a gardener—to set up the right conditions. The same holds true for ChiRunning. Your job is to learn to set up the optimal conditions for chi to move through your body, and voilà . . . running happens!

THE CHIRUNNING METHOD

Here are the optimal conditions for efficient running and the fundamentals of the ChiRunning method:

- Great posture
- Relaxed limbs
- Loose joints
- Engaged core muscles
- A focused mind
- Good breathing technique

Here are some of the benefits of using the ChiRunning method:

- Great posture
- Relaxed limbs
- Loose joints
- Engaged core muscles
- A focused mind
- Good breathing technique
- More energy

You see? The *process* is the goal! There are many more great benefits of ChiRunning, but I just want to make the point that the ChiRunning method is holistic, which means that each of the components of the technique contributes positively to the whole by supporting the others to do their job. This aspect of the ChiRunning method also ensures that you don't have to become an expert in all of the components right away. I've had clients benefit enormously from just one hour of learning how to improve their posture. Any single component will benefit your running, and when all of the components are working together, the effects can be nothing short of transformational.

Unlike power running, it's hard to imagine that one could get injured from doing anything on this list. None of these fundamentals will injure you. And because it's virtually impossible to overdo any of them, there is not a downside.

As you learn to incorporate the ChiRunning method into your running you will dramatically reduce your dependence on strong leg muscles. Gravity will be pulling you forward and your speed will be a function of your ability to relax more deeply, not your ability to push harder. I call it "smart effort."

Personally, I really don't have any huge desire to spend endless hours building and maintaining muscles, drinking protein shakes to feed those hungry muscles, and taking ibuprofen to relieve sore muscles . . . so I've decided to work my *mind* instead.

THE CHIRUNNING MIND-SET

The ChiRunning mind-set teaches you to listen and focus internally rather than on arbitrary, external goals. The mind-set of ChiRunning is based on consistently establishing a clear link of communication between your mind and your body, whereby the process becomes the goal. Your body becomes both your teacher and your pupil. If you pay close attention to it, you'll come to know what it can and can't do. With that knowledge, you can then teach it new skills and habits. The place to begin is to feel and see what's going on in your body at any given time, and then respond accordingly in the moment. It is called Body Sensing, and I will tell you more about this skill in Chapter 3. ChiRunning teaches you to be a master of your own body and your own best coach.

There is such cultural pressure in our society to be athletic and have a perfect body. I encounter many people with a negative self-image because they don't see themselves as an athlete, even though they might walk or run four days a week. This negative self-image stops people from listening to the messages their bodies are trying to convey. As I watch beginning runners study their own movement and make necessary corrections to inefficient movements, I can often see the smile of self-confidence spreading across their face.

Shirlee, 56, like many of my clients, has always felt bad about herself because she breathes hard when she runs. She was so embarrassed about her heavy breathing, she wasn't able to focus in class. When she finally confided in me, I was able to give her some tools that helped her to breathe more efficiently. Now her focus is on breathing correctly instead of being embarrassed!

The ChiRunning mind-set is like a dance between your mind and your body—a delightfully cooperative tango. There is a clear, two-way conversation happening all the time between the partners—a constant flow in the moment to create the best conditions for harmonious movement. The ChiRunning mind-set involves not only practicing to connect your mind with your body, it also involves using that connection as a way to respond to any challenging circumstances that might come your way, such as uphills, downhills, trails, adverse weather or surface conditions, mile 18 of a marathon, fatigue, or anything else that may be perceived as an impediment to your forward movement. ChiRunning is a toolkit for your mind and body to respond to whatever is coming at you.

COOPERATING WITH TWO FORCES: THE FORCE OF GRAVITY AND THE FORCE OF THE ROAD

Let the Force be with you. —OBI-WAN KENOBI

In T'ai Chi one of the first things we are taught is that the best way to deal with a force is to cooperate with it, not oppose it. If you go *against* a force, you give it more power. On the other hand, if you move in the *same* direction of a force (cooperation), you neutralize its power. If you want to respond correctly to any force, learn to be receptive; the force can become your friend, and possibly even your ally.

Whenever you're running, your body comes under the influence of two forces acting on it: the constant downward pull of gravity, and the force of the road coming at you as you move forward. In ChiRunning we learn to cooperate and make these forces allies with every step, and good posture is the main ingredient for handling both.

THE PULL OF GRAVITY

The pull of gravity is a big force that can either assist you in moving down the road (if you cooperate) or cause you to work harder (if you don't cooperate). Here's the science behind this statement. Anytime you run with your body upright (as in power running) your center of mass is located directly over your feet and your posture is in alignment with the downward pull of gravity. Standing in this position is an example of Newton's first law of motion: "A body at rest tends to stay at rest unless acted upon by an external force." In this position your body is at rest and won't move unless *you* move it by pushing yourself forward with your legs, which is why we call it power running in the first place. Then, as soon as you stop pushing yourself forward, you stop moving. All of your motion is dependent on you, and because you are pushing yourself off the ground to move forward, you're working against gravity.

With the ChiRunning technique, instead of holding your posture upright and in line with the pull of gravity, you allow yourself to cooperate *with* the pull of gravity by letting yourself fall forward. Your body will then become a forward-falling object (like a tree that's just been chopped down). Because your center of mass (your pelvis) is just ahead of your point of contact with the ground (your feet), your upper body falls forward . . . and all you have to do is pick up your feet to keep up with your fall (see figures 3 and 4 on the next page).

When you learn to balance yourself in this slight forward lean, you'll be cooperating with the same force that pulls a unicycle rider forward. So if gravity is pulling you, just *go with it* and you'll be running more efficiently than you ever imagined. All of those poor, overworked lower leg muscles can take the day off because they are no longer needed for pushing. Can you imagine how good your legs would feel if they were used *only* for momentary support between strides and didn't have to be used for propulsion?

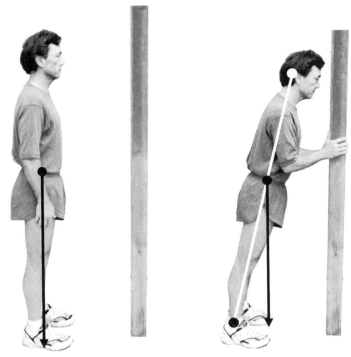

Figure 3—Center of mass upright   **Figure 4—Center of mass leaning**

THE FORCE OF THE ROAD

Here's how to cooperate with the other force you'll be dealing with: the force of the road coming at you. Whenever your body moves forward, the road is always moving in the *opposite* direction at the same speed, relatively speaking. Most power runners reach forward with their legs and land with a heel strike in front of their body. If you reach forward with your legs when you run, you are actually swinging *into* the force of the road coming at you and more often than not your heel will hit the ground in front of you. It's like a mini head-on collision between your foot and the road. The impact of a heel strike can send a shock wave up your leg, potentially damaging your heels, ankles, shins, knees, hips, or lower back, depending on where your weakest link lies. Having your foot strike in front of your body is, in fact, the same as putting on the brakes because your feet are basically stopping your forward momentum each time they hit the ground.

Pretty inefficient, I'd say. If you don't believe me, just look at the bottoms of your shoes and check to see if the heels are worn down. Those are your "brake pads."

So, if you're power running with an upright body position, you're pushing yourself forward with one leg while you're putting the brakes on with the other leg. What's wrong with this picture? Would you ever drive your car with one foot on the gas pedal and one foot on the brake pedal at the same time?

With the ChiRunning technique, we'll show you how to land with your foot slightly behind your center of mass, so that your center of mass is *in front* of your point of contact. This allows your legs to swing out *behind you* without adding a braking component to your stride. Instead of landing with a heel strike, you'll land with a nice soft *midfoot* strike, and all the force of the road coming at you will pass on by without slowing you down or impacting your body. When you're leading with your upper body and relaxing your lower body, the force of the road coming your way will *swing your legs for you*. All the lower body focuses in Chapter 4 are designed to help you cooperate with the force of the road and make it your ally.

Make Your Running a Practice

A new idea we'd like to further with the advent of ChiRunning is something running has needed for a long time: that is, to be transformed from a sport to a practice. Think about it. If you see running only as a sport, you're limiting yourself to getting only the physical benefits. It's like the difference between stretching and yoga . . . between sitting in a waiting room and sitting in meditation . . . between training your body to run faster or farther and practicing to run in a mindful and masterful way.

Making an activity a practice is a process of self-mastery. You are no longer simply practicing that activity; you use it to learn about, understand, and master yourself as well as the activity. In ChiRunning you have the opportunity not just to keep physically fit without injury but also to learn about and master your body, observe and focus your mind, and, yes, even become more aware of and free your spirit.

One reason to practice a skill is to make that skill easier until it doesn't take effort. Think about it. If you practice playing a violin, every time you practice, your goal is to get to know the instrument better so it becomes easier to play. You practice your scales so you can add fluidity to your fingering and play notes quickly. When you practice yoga, you work toward creating flexibility and strength in your mind and body, with greater ease. When you regularly practice meditation, you find a quiet and focused mind more readily, even when your day is stressful. When you practice your golf swing, that perfect connection with the ball occurs more often.

When you make your running a practice it becomes a vehicle for personal growth as well as fitness. A practice is a regular, mindful activity that works to enhance your quality of life. A good practice will help your body, emotions, mind, and spirit evolve and progress. Part of the ChiRunning practice is to become a good listener, a good student, and a good practitioner of what you learn.

Here is what a few clients have said:

"From the single clinic I did with you I have grown immensely. Through what I learned in your clinic, I am in essence learning to walk again, and learning to run again, and the new ease I am finding there is continuing to spill over into all other aspects of my life."

—Darryl Denton, age 54

"I'm amazed and thrilled by your teachings and have already started straightening my spine as I sit and walk. Good posture is my new mantra."

—Patrick Nolan, age 37

When you make ChiRunning a practice, it can become more than just a sport because it engages your mind and creates a stronger connection with your body, while improving the health of your whole body.

DISCOVERY AND UNFOLDMENT

One of the great joys of teaching ChiRunning is seeing people experience running, and themselves, in a way they never imagined. Time and time again people have expressed sheer wonder and amazement at how great they feel running. From people who were told they could never run again to complete beginners with little self-confidence, to accomplished runners looking to improve their race times, ChiRunning has had great results.

It works because all of the underlying principles are based on moving within the laws of Nature. When you learn to listen to your body, nothing is forced and everything progresses as it should, with little disruption. Ultimately, this approach to running, based on self-discovery and the natural unfoldment of your potential, offers one an opportunity to develop a richer relationship to one's body and Being.

ChiRunning takes you into new territory where running is no longer externally driven but internally motivated. The emphasis is no longer on running increased speeds or distances, because those become by-products of sound, efficient running form. But you speed demons out there can rest assured that there need be no sacrifice in speed or distance; in fact, it's quite the opposite, if you're so inclined. You can run faster and farther than ever with less effort *and* little or no harm to your body. And what about those of you who aren't speed demons? Well, you can simply enjoy being a self-respecting athlete at any age or any skill level. The goal is to be able to run freely and joyfully for the rest of your life, and for you to enjoy the full range of benefits that running offers—physically, mentally . . . and, yes, spiritually.

CHAPTER TWO

The Principles of ChiRunning: Moving with Nature

Principles are deep fundamental truths that have universal application. Principles are guidelines for human conduct that are proven to have enduring, permanent value.
—STEPHEN COVEY

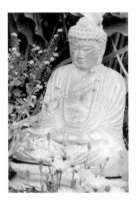

ChiRunning is based on a set of principles that will help you run, and train, in a more effortless and efficient way. These principles are a huge part of my regular T'ai Chi lessons with Master Xu and have had a profound impact on me, not only in how I move my body but also in how I understand the world and, in turn, guide my life.

Thousands of years ago, Chinese masters studied how Nature works and defined these principles in writings such as the *Tao Te Ching* (the most widely translated book besides the Bible) and the *I Ching* (the preeminent book of Chinese philosophy) and in the practice of T'ai Chi (the mother of martial arts). But it's not just the Chinese who have studied these principles. Guys like Einstein and Newton defined many of them as the laws of physics.

It is no wonder people of deep wisdom and intellect chose to study

Nature. It has a set of basic principles that seem to work pretty well. Anyone can see how perfectly Nature operates when left to itself. Everything in Nature has a deep sense of order and rightness. It is harmonious. You don't find animals out of place, and plants don't grow where the conditions are not right. Even on the molecular level, everything has an order and a place, and somehow it's all held in balance. It all works!

These laws can also be thought of as universal laws. For a law to be universal, it has to hold true on all four basic levels of existence: physical, emotional, mental, and spiritual. For instance, one law says, "A body at rest tends to remain at rest unless acted upon by an external force."

Here are some examples of how this law works on different levels:

- **On the physical level:** A couch potato won't move unless the power goes off and the TV goes blank or he runs out of chips.
- **On the mental level:** It's a philosophical change, such as when Christopher Columbus came along and discovered the New World.
- **On an emotional level:** I can go through an entire day absorbed in my own drama until my daughter throws her arms around my neck and says, "I love you, Daddy," which zaps me out of my brain and into my heart.
- **On a spiritual level:** It might take a near-death experience for someone to realize how precious life really is.

The beauty of universal laws is that when you learn a law on one level, it can show you how life works on other levels.

WHAT HAPPENS WHEN YOU RESIST OR DON'T FOLLOW THE LAW?

Well, I can pretty safely say the consequence of breaking a universal law is more than just paying a fine and promising not to do it again. It will increase your workload in the short term and will inevitably lead to some level of failure in the long term. In your running, you may have more speed, but you'll have a beat-up body. You may have a good race but feel like hell the next day. Working against the laws of physics requires you to rely more on your own strength than on the forces of Nature.

Running can be in harmony with the laws of nature, but power running is not. The fact that there are more than 16 million injuries in the United States annually should be cause for alarm. No wonder *Sports Injury Bulletin* classifies running as a high-injury sport. The questions that this brings up are: (1) Should people be running? (2) Is there a better way?

For question 1, the answer is yes. Our physiology is well suited for running. We were designed to run. As for question 2, from my own experience with ChiRunning and having taught it to thousands of people, I can say unequivocally that yes, there is a better way.

Have you ever tried to swim upstream? You can do it if you're strong enough. And if you're not strong enough, you can work hard and build big muscles so that you can eventually do it. But no matter how you look at it, you're swimming against the current, and that's going to take a lot of work. I mean, salmon do it, but they die when they get there. So as long as you're in the water, you have to follow the law of the water. On the other hand, if you want to get upstream with less effort, simply get out of the water and into a different set of laws, where getting upstream might involve nothing more than a gentle walk up a fern-lined path. As Cecil B. DeMille said regarding his epic film *The Ten Commandments*, "It is impossible for us to break the law ourselves. We can only break ourselves against the law."

Going with the Flow

When you are working within natural laws, there is less effort involved and less of the physical breakdown experienced with power running. When you run economically, you don't require as much fuel to keep going, you don't get tired as easily, and it doesn't take as long to recover from your runs. When you are not overworking your muscles and joints, there will be less chance for injury. When you cooperate with universal law, you become powerful on all levels, including attitude. You will be able to go out for a run and come back feeling better than when you took off. When you integrate the laws of Nature into your consciousness, you can learn how to use them in your running, or in your life, to *create the conditions for energy to flow.*

THE KEY PRINCIPLES

Here are the key principles on which ChiRunning is based. In this chapter I'll go over their definitions, and in Chapter 4 I'll apply these principles to very specific focuses and exercises that will help you move your body in a more fluid, efficient, and graceful way, one step at a time. There are many more than three principles that guide the movement of Nature, but we have used these particular principles specifically to benefit your running. The three key principles are:

1. Needle in Cotton: alignment and relaxation
2. Gradual Progress: the step-by-step approach
3. Balance in Motion: physical balance and complementary balance

As you become more adept at practicing and integrating these principles into your running, you will begin to feel an ease in how your body moves. Instead of your body being a tool for running, your running becomes a tool for your body.

NEEDLE IN COTTON: ALIGNMENT AND RELAXATION

This is one of the main principles taught in T'ai Chi. It is considered the foundation of all movement in the body. The phrase "needle in cotton" describes the feeling that a T'ai Chi practitioner should have while doing the form. You align your body and concentrate chi energy to your center, while your arms and legs are as soft as cotton, holding no tension.

Here's the image. Think of a needle held vertically inside of a ball of cotton. The needle represents your centerline, your axis of rotation when running. The needle is very "gathered," as the Chinese would say. It represents the gathering of energy toward a center. It is thin and straight and strong, which is how you want your posture line to be whenever you're moving through space. As you gather energy toward your centerline, you draw it away from your peripherals, leaving them as soft as cotton. In ChiRunning, as in T'ai Chi, all movement in your body originates in your center. It is your power source, acting as the axis around which everything else moves. According to T'ai Chi, your center, or *dan tien*, is located just below your navel and in front of your spine. It is conveniently hooked up to your arms and legs by a series of bones, ligaments, and tendons, so whenever you move your center, your arms and legs move too. But in order for your center to do its work efficiently, your spine (needle) has to be aligned to allow for free rotation of your trunk, and all the moving parts of your body (arms, legs, shoulders, and hips) must be as soft as cotton (flexible and relaxed) in order to move freely and not work against any motion created by your center.

The emphasis in ChiRunning is on learning how to run from your center, and the better you get at that, the less you depend on your legs to run. I know that sounds counterintuitive, but it's true. When Master Xu is teaching me to move, he has me gather my energy and mental focus into my *dan tien* while softening the rest of my body so that it will be moved by my center and not by my muscles. When I move in this way, I can feel the fluidity in my gait led by the movement in my center. It takes the emphasis away from my legs, allowing them to become secondary in my movement.

When you run from a place outside your center, it is less powerful because you are doing so from an unbalanced state. Your legs have to work many times harder than if the rest of your body were helping out. When you don't run from your center, your running form is not organized, because your arms and legs and trunk are moving as three independent entities instead of one harmonious, fluid unit. I have observed many runners who are moving their arms and legs and going through the motions of running, but what is missing is the sense of integrity that comes from having a strong center.

Our Milky Way has a center around which all the stars in the galaxy rotate. Our solar system has a center, the sun, around which all the planets rotate. Our earth also has a center, and it spins on an axis that runs right through it. Our country has a center that is said to be somewhere in Missouri, although I've never been there. In the ChiRunning technique, it all begins by learning to locate and sense your center when you run.

Try this: Stand up straight, with your best posture and one foot slightly behind the other, hip width apart. Relax your shoulders and let your arms hang limp at your sides. Now pretend that your spine is a vertical axle. Let it rotate first in one direction and then in the other. As you rotate your spine back and forth, your arms will move because your spine is moving; let them flail against your body in a gentle way. Focus on keeping your spine straight while rotating back and forth. Stay with the image of your spine being an axle. Try to see how relaxed you can make your shoulders, arms, and wrists. This is an example of your core doing the work while your arms are just along for the ride.

Here is a visualization to practice anytime during the day and as often as possible. Imagine a line between the top of your head and your tailbone. This is your centerline. Keep it in your mind's eye when you are walking or running. Start by focusing on it while you're standing still. Become friends with it and remember it. Make it as familiar as your breath. Don't try to do anything with it. Just acknowledge it. See it. Learn that it is a location within your body.

Find your center in your body.
Sense your center in your feelings.
See your center in your mind.
Be centered in your spirit.

GRADUAL PROGRESS: THE STEP-BY-STEP APPROACH

The Gradual Progress principle says that everything has to grow incrementally through its own developmental stages, from less to more or from smaller to larger. When a growth process happens gradually, each step forms a stable foundation for the next step. This principle holds true for any growth process, whether it's an object, an idea, a feeling, or a life-form. An example on the physical plane would be a tree growing from a seed. It starts off small and gets larger as the cells divide and multiply. Another example would be a business start-up. The owner begins a business from an idea that develops into a plan that leads to opening its doors to the public. The business world start off small, and if the owner did things right, it would grow into a thriving enterprise.

If you try to break this law and skip steps, you'll encounter either a negative effect on the process or a diminished outcome. Consider the terminal torrid love affair, in which two people meet and instantly have the hots for each other. They spend the next four nights joined at the hip and then skip off to Las Vegas to get married. Then they file for a divorce after about three weeks because they forgot to build a friendship.

As you may have already guessed, a big factor in the success of this principle is time. Lots of people come to me and say they'd like to run a marathon. The first question I ask them is, "How long is your current long run?" If they answer with a distance under 10K, my next question is, "Which year would you like to run it?" Running a marathon is not that hard to do if you take plenty of time to slowly improve your running technique and build up your mileage. The first race I ever trained for and ran was a 50-mile race. That may seem really far for a first race, and it was. But I trained for three and a half years to do it. I started off with a long run of 10 miles and increased my mileage only when it felt right. Building up slowly allowed my body to adjust to the increasing mileage. It allowed me to take the time to correct imperfections in my form that were causing me pain. But most of all, it allowed me to gradually build the confidence that running 50 miles didn't have to be a big deal or harmful to my body.

I witness runners breaking this rule most often on race day. Everyone lines up at the starting line, and when the gun fires, they take off as if the finish line were at the end of the block. If I stick around for the finish of the race, I usually see the familiar faces of those rabbits who shot away from the starting line, only now they look a little like a bad guy in a western movie, staggering forward after being shot in the back.

This scenario happens a lot in power running. The basic script is:

(1) train hard for the race; (2) once you start the race, run as fast as you can and hang on to whatever speed you can until your fuel runs out; (3) try to get across the finish line without losing that bagel you slam-dunked on your way out of the house.

The principle of Gradual Progress is always applied in ChiRunning, whether it's a single run or a running program. When starting a run, it's important to start slowly and pick up the speed as your body adapts to the movement of running. Just as you wouldn't drive off from a stoplight in fourth gear, you wouldn't start a run too fast. Instead, you accelerate through the gears until you reach your cruising speed. Your body is no exception. Don't start a running program with too much speed or mileage or you could get injured. Most training injuries happen when someone's ego starts getting ahead of the rate at which his body can produce new muscle cells. For something to end up solid, it has to grow step-by-step and move through all of the sequential stages of growth. If you start skipping steps, you're breaking this law, and the consequences can range from fatigue to aches to injuries. Sixty percent of all running injuries occur because of overtraining, which means either too much mileage or too fast an upgrade in speed or mileage. On the emotional level, if you start off a program too fast and burn out because of the intensity, you could end up not even wanting to go out and run. I'll use this principle extensively in Chapter 6, "Program Development."

If I break this law when I'm running, I pay in one form or another: I end up with a slower time, sore legs, longer recovery, or even injury. When I start off too fast with an activity in my life, I increase my odds of failure or disappointment. Go step-by-step, gradually increase, and let each new stage be built on what you've learned from the preceding stages. Gradual Progress—it's a law we can live with.

Balance in Motion:
Complementary Balance and Physical Balance

You've probably seen the symbol for yin/yang. It's a circle that is half black and half white, with an S-shaped line separating the two halves. Among other things, it is the symbol of balance. But unlike a circle with a line straight down the middle, dividing the figure into two equal halves, the shape represents complementary energy balance. Notice that as one portion of the circle gets larger, the section of the circle on the other side of the line gets smaller. Whenever one side is expanded, the other side is contracted. When one side is hard, one side is soft. When one side is light, the other side is heavy. When something is active, something else has to be receptive. Balance doesn't always mean equal balance. It means that when two complementary forces are interacting in relatively good measure, there is a state of balance and centeredness.

In your running, you need to be balanced in two ways: balanced in your *effort* and balanced in your *physical movement.* In ChiRunning, as in T'ai Chi, the physical balance happens in six directions: left to right, up to down, and front to back. As one part of your body moves forward, its complement moves to the rear. As your body leans forward, your stride opens up behind you. Whenever one side of your body is extending, the other side is gathering. You're always trying to create symmetry in how your body moves by not emphasizing either your left or right side. Your upper body usage is balanced with your lower body usage.

If you run with just your legs, without bringing in all the help from the rest of the body, then you're running in an unbalanced state, and your legs will be overworked. If you have a heavy rock to move, it's much easier to get five people to do it so the workload gets spread out. ChiRunning is a way to run with all of your body engaged in a unified way, each part doing its proportional share. When all parts are working in harmony, your body moves in a balanced way. When a cheetah runs, there is no part of its body that isn't contributing to the effort, and its running is balanced.

The key to finding balance is to know where your center is so that you can be balanced around it. When you check to see whether your body is in balance, compare your right side to your left side. Is one of your shoulders higher than the other? Does one foot turn out? The middle point is your centerline, and you want each side of the centerline to be in balance. In Chapter 4 we'll help you create balance in your whole body so that your running is in balance and therefore more efficient.

Here are a few examples of how balance can manifest itself:

- Balance of fluids: The more you sweat, the more you need to drink.
- Balance of workouts: Alternate easy and hard workouts.
- Balance of fuel: The harder you work, the more fuel you require.
- Balance of effort: The faster you run, the more you need to relax your legs.
- Balance of work and play: The harder you work, the more important it is that you play.

Until we learn to move in a way where we cooperate with the laws of Nature, our forward progress will forever be met with resistance in the form of injury, fatigue, disappointment, or plain old difficulty. When you allow yourself to be guided by these principles, running becomes a way to create health for your whole being, and any doubts about whether or not running is good for you will evaporate. With the power of Nature backing you up, the potential for success and enjoyment is vast.

CHAPTER THREE

The Four Chi-Skills

> How do you best move toward mastery? To put it simply, you practice diligently, but you practice primarily *for the sake of the practice itself.* —GEORGE LEONARD, *MASTERY*

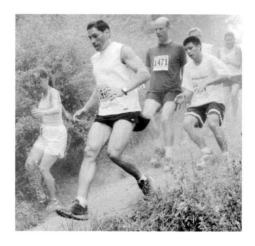

I spent fifteen years as a woodworker, learning the value of always working to improve one's skill level. Whenever I made a costly miscalculation, I was forced to call on ingenuity and skill to pull me out of the fire. I can honestly say that I learned more skills from the countless mistakes I made than from all the woodworking books on my shelf. I was also blessed to have some highly talented mentors teaching me the resourcefulness to turn a tree into a finely crafted piece of furniture.

Craftsmen and artisans depend on their skills to see them through any challenge that might arise. It is no different with running, or with life, for that matter. My two seemingly disparate fields of interest share the same four underlying skills, which I call Chi-Skills: Focusing, Body Sensing, Breathing, and Relaxing.

The Chi-Skills are my essential tools for running that I'd like to share with you. There is no question that when I run a 50K race, I am using all of these skills to maximize performance while minimizing physical effort. The use of Chi-Skills allows your running to become multidimensional. Your workouts will have more depth and breadth because there's something more going on than running. You will begin to approach running in ways that go beyond the realms of farther or faster.

These skills will help you reach any goal in life with greater ease. Although we all use them every day, we often do so unconsciously. By consciously practicing Chi-Skills in your running, you will increase your capacity to focus your mind, sense your body, relax (don't most of us have trouble with this important skill?), and maximize the benefits of the most basic of acts—breathing.

As always in ChiRunning, the process is the goal. Chi-Skills are both valuable skills and worthwhile goals at the same time. So, every time you practice focusing your mind, you are accomplishing your goal of being more focused. It is a very satisfying effort.

In Chapter 6 we will go into details of how to incorporate the Chi-Skills and the technique focuses into your running program. But for now, practicing any of these skills for five minutes on a run, or while doing practically anything else (from washing dishes to changing a diaper), will increase your capability with that skill and also improve the caliber of your run or activity. These skills improve the quality of your running *and* the quality of your life.

Focusing Your Mind

ChiRunning is the thinking person's way to run. There will never be a *ChiRunning for Dummies*. Although it's important for people to get a physical experience first, it is the mind that really does the bulk of the work in ChiRunning. Your mind turns off the chatter and focuses so it can listen to your body. Your mind instructs your muscles to start working or relaxing. Your mind orchestrates the perfect run, starting out slowly, finding the perfect tempo, and taking in the beauty and chi of your surroundings so that you finish relaxed, empowered, and full of energy for the day ahead.

There are many worthwhile reasons to learn something new, whether it's ChiRunning, a foreign language, a musical instrument, or a new recipe. Learning is what we are meant to do. It is our birthright as humans. If we stop learning, we stop growing and our minds become stagnant. If you don't use it, you'll lose it.

Two of the key ingredients (and great benefits) of learning and practicing ChiRunning are *a focused mind* and *a responsive body*. Being able to use your mind to direct the movements of your body is a big step toward the physical mastery of any activity. The ChiRunning focuses are designed to train your mind to sense, respond to, and direct the movements of your body when you're running, standing, sitting, or walking.

USING YOUR Y'CHI

When your mind is used to direct the energy and movement of your body *through your eyes*, you're using what the Chinese call *y'chi* (pronounced "ee-chee"), a full mind/body focus and a great skill to have if you want to improve your efficiency and speed. It's the unbreakable focus of a bird dog on point, a tennis player awaiting a serve, or a meter maid while she's writing you a parking ticket.

It is best to understand y'chi with the example of a cat hunting its prey. I'm sure you've seen a cat that has just spotted a nearby bird. The cat fixes its gaze on its prey and seems to become frozen in place. Then, without breaking its gaze, the cat begins to slowly and quietly creep toward the bird in a motion that can only be described as "a cat doing T'ai Chi." Its limbs are soft and its feet seem to be touching the ground ever so softly, so as to not make a sound. The one thing that doesn't change is the visual contact the cat keeps with the bird. That's y'chi. The visual focus of the cat is informing the cat's body how to move. It's not a thought process for the cat. The cat's y'chi is what is "pulling" the cat toward the bird.

All the great athletes utilize y'chi whether they know it or not. In soccer the players never take their eyes off the ball. In hockey it's the puck. In baseball . . . you get the idea. When Tiger Woods stands over his golf ball, he first looks at his goal and then looks down at the ball, and before he begins his swing, he gathers all the focus he can muster on all levels. Then, while holding all that focus, he begins his swing and does not take his eyes off the ball until his club makes contact with it. That's y'chi . . . and it happens when *everything* is aligned: your body, your vision, your forward movement, your mind, *and* your heart.

Practicing your y'chi will always leave you feeling energized and clearheaded because your mind becomes so focused on your goal. When you can maintain unbroken visual contact with an object or goal, it leaves little room for your mind to be doing any of its normal antics of following every thought that comes into your consciousness. I'll explain exactly how to practice your y'chi in Chapter 4.

"But who wants to focus that much?" you might ask. "I just run to relax and rest my mind." Like a meditation practice, the training of the mind and body in ChiRunning is more relaxing than letting the mind wander. Studies have shown that watching TV is not as relaxing as sitting quietly. A focused mind is more relaxed than a mind that wanders aimlessly through the details and minutiae of the day. When you are focused on teaching yourself something new, the benefits to your body and mind will far outweigh the effort it takes to focus. Eventually, as the ChiRunning form becomes second nature, your mind and body become as one. It is no longer *work* to focus your mind. It is not even a thought process, because the situation and the response are simultaneous. Like the cat stalking the bird, you're pulled forward by your y'chi. Practicing the ChiRunning focuses is preparation for developing and utilizing your y'chi in any situation.

Bob, age 48, had been a recreational runner for fifteen years when he came to his first ChiRunning class. He told me that he had gone out five days a week for the past three years and run a 3-mile loop around his neighborhood like clockwork. He had done it so regularly that he knew within seconds how long it would take him to arrive back at his own front door. After attending the ChiRunning clinic, he went out the next day, armed with all of the focuses that he could remember, and proceeded to run his loop as usual. He was used to coming home feeling a distinct sense of having done his obligatory exercise for the day. This day, when he arrived back at his house, he looked at his watch, expecting to see the usual numbers. To his surprise, his time was 3 minutes faster than his previous best. He told me he thought his watch had stopped during the run, so he tapped on it to make sure it was working. Not only that, he wasn't at all tired. In fact, he felt so good that he immediately went out and ran another 2 miles! He had done so well at keeping his mind attentive to the focuses that his body could simply relax and go along for the ride!

Keeping the ChiRunning focuses can be a meditative practice that trains your mind to curtail its arbitrary wanderings. As in meditation, the greater aspect of ChiRunning is that you learn how to be present with your mind and body, which is where true inner freedom lies.

If all you want to do is learn to run without injuring yourself, or perhaps get a little faster or run longer, ChiRunning can get you there. If you're also interested in the benefits of meditation and the power of a focused mind, ChiRunning can offer you that as well. For it is a focused mind moving with the relaxed, responsive body that does, in the end, give you the ease of movement you're looking for.

If you'd like a sample of what it feels like to focus your mind, try this: Sit up straight in your chair and hold your best posture while you read the rest of this chapter. Don't let yourself slouch even once. That's it! Your focus is to maintain good posture. I'll ask you at the end of this chapter how you did.

BODY SENSING: HIGH-SPEED ACCESS

Of all the Chi-Skills, Body Sensing is the most important. Without the ability to sense when you're moving your body either correctly or incorrectly, you'll be dead in the water in terms of improving your running technique. Having the ability to clearly sense the nuances of how your body is moving will allow you to make the adjustments necessary to improving your efficiency and reducing your exertion level at any speed.

Body Sensing is the skill of having your mind and your body working together as a team. The more you practice building a clear communication link between your mind and your body, the quicker your running will grow into a new level of ease and joy.

When I was a kid, my brother and I used to play telephone with two tin cans and a piece of wire. It was a primitive mode of communication, but it worked. Now I have a computer with a cable modem, and I can send e-mail, music, and photos. There are many methods available today, but the underlying theme is to improve our ability to communicate.

The tin cans have many parallels to Body Sensing. When I first started to run, many years ago, it was on the tin-can level: My *mind* would tell my body to go out and run. Then I would run until my *body* said it was tired, which would then trigger my mind to call it quits for the day. That was the extent of the communication between my body and my mind.

Now that I'm more skilled at Body Sensing, I can carefully listen to the subtle nuances of my running form and make small adjustments in the moment. Each time I make an adjustment, I listen very carefully with my mind to what my body is saying. I never judge my body's responses as good or bad. They're just responses, and I'm collecting data. At this point my mind and body communicate more intuitively, like an old married couple. I not only enjoy the interaction, I depend on it. If I listen carefully enough, my body will tell me everything I need to know to create optimal results.

Here is another tin-can analogy. When I talked to my brother through that primitive wire connection, there was usually so much static on the line that I could barely make out what he was saying. If the wire touched any obstacles between him and me, additional noise would come through the line and garble the message. Likewise, there are factors that will add "static" to your line, making it difficult to receive a clear message from your body. The static that I'm talking about is generated by your mental activity—your ideas and attitudes about what your body is doing or could be doing. Body Sensing is not a *thinking* process, it's a *sensing* process. Watch for phrases like "I should" or "I can't" or "I'm not" or "I have to." Any negative or judgmental thinking creates static on the line. And who needs that when you're trying to get clear reception?

Body Sensing is the skill I have used in the *process* of learning and developing ChiRunning, and it has also become a skill that is now second nature.

The ChiRunning technique is more than just a running form. It is an activity that works to build a strong link between your mind and body. When learning the ChiRunning technique, you will be asked to move your body in a particular way and then to Body Sense so you can tell if what you're doing is effective.

HOW TO BODY SENSE

This is one of my favorite exercises for learning Body Sensing. You will learn how to tell the difference between perception and reality when it comes to your body—a skill we could all use.

Exercise: The Mirror Exercise

1. Stand in front of a full-length mirror. Keeping your eyes closed, position yourself with your feet parallel, your knees slightly bent, shoulders squared, arms and hands relaxed at your sides.
2. Begin by sensing your feet on the ground and the position your feet are in. Feel your legs. Feel your hips. Feel your torso . . . your arms, hands, shoulders, and the position of your head.

   Imagine how you look by how your body feels to you. Spend time really feeling the position of your body.
3. After one minute of doing this, open your eyes. Note all the differences between how you *thought* your body looked and how your body actually looks in the mirror.

   - Are your feet truly parallel?
   - Are your shoulders aligned with each other?
   - Are your fingers straight or curved?
   - Is your head on straight?

Now stand sideways to the mirror and close your eyes again. Make your feet parallel and stand with your best posture. Again, take one minute to really feel the position of your body. When you open your eyes, you'll have to turn your head and look at yourself from the side. Once again, note the differences between what you felt and what you see in the mirror.

   - Is your spine vertical or slumped?
   - Is your chin up or down?

Practice this regularly, and you'll become adept at truly sensing the positions of your arms, legs, and body. You'll also become more skilled at directing your body to move as you want it to move.

This exercise is similar to what goes on when I videotape students. They'll think they're running in a certain way, but when they see what they're actually doing, it has a huge impact on their view of themselves. Seeing the "truth" through the eyes of a video camera allows them to make adjustments with a much greater degree of accuracy.

Do this mirror exercise first thing every morning before your day really gets rolling, or whenever you're at the gym. The entire exercise should take less than five minutes. The longer it takes, the better it will work for you. Don't hurry through it; take the time to enjoy sensing your body and getting to know it. Faster is not better. Doing this exercise consistently will build your ability to sense what is going on anywhere in your body.

THE 3 STEPS TO BODY SENSING

Here's a more general how-to of Body Sensing in three steps. Try to get a sense of what each step means for you. They're guidelines for how to develop the skill of Body Sensing. You can repeat these steps as many times as needed to affect change.

1. **Listen carefully.** Whenever you make an adjustment to your running form practice listening to any little nuances that you can detect. How is your body moving, and what does it feel like? What sensations are you noticing in various parts?
2. **Assess the information.** Ask yourself if your body is moving in the way you intend it to. Do your best to discern if any adjustment you're trying to apply is working or not. If it feels easier then try to memorize that sensation and how you got there. If its more difficult or uncomfortable then try to sense what doesn't feel quite right.
3. **Adjust incrementally**. Making subtle adjustments is always the best policy. Any abrupt change in how you move your body is an invitation for injury.

In Chapter 4 you will be learning how to use your mind to set up the ChiRunning Form Focuses which are the building blocks of sound, efficient technique. As you work with each of these focuses, you will have to Body Sense whether or not you are doing them correctly. Let's say that your focus is to relax your ankles while you run. First, your mind will tell your ankles to relax. Then you will feel your ankles to see if they are indeed relaxing. If you do it right, your ankles will feel soft and loose, in which case you will memorize what it feels like to have relaxed ankles so you can remember how to relax them the next time you go running. If you don't fully relax your ankles, you might sense a pulling in your Achilles tendon or tightness in your calves. That's your body telling you that relaxation isn't happening. So you go back and ask your ankles to make the adjustment again. It's best to repeat this cycle until you feel satisfied that you're moving correctly, or at least in the right direction.

When you're first learning Body Sensing, it is invaluable to have someone videotape you while you run. Then you can play back the tape and either stop the action or slow it down to see every detail of how you're moving. This will allow you to make a direct comparison between what you were attempting to do and what you are actually doing. You may think you are leaning when you're not. You may think that your arms are swinging like crazy when they're just hanging at your sides. People have their biggest breakthroughs when they see themselves on video. This is because they can remember how they *felt* when they were running, then match that up with how they *looked* in the video.

THE BODY SCAN

Another important Body Sensing tool is the Body Scan. You can do Body Scans regularly; in the morning when you get up, during the day, and especially before, during, and after a run. Make it a regular habit.

Start at your head and work your way down your body. All you have to do is focus your attention on each area and see if you sense any tenseness, stiffness, discomfort, or pain. If you don't, send up a prayer of thanks and move on. If you feel something that doesn't seem right, focus your mind on that area and take a deep breath. Try to relax the area if it's tense or stiff. Move it around or shake it and let go of any tension.

If you come upon an area that needs lots of help, do a little and then move on to the rest of your body. After you've relaxed and loosened all the other areas, you can come back to the "biggie" and give it some special attention.

The following is a sequential list of areas of your body. To familiarize yourself with each of these areas, start at the top of the list. As you move through the list place your hands on any body parts you can't easily sense. The touch will facilitate connecting your mind with that part of your body. Pause in each location for a few seconds and see if you can feel any tension or soreness. Then move on through the list, pausing at each area to listen. If you're reading this book and sitting in a chair, don't get up. You can do this one sitting down.

Sense   your . . . Head . . . Neck . . . Shoulders . . . Arms . . . Elbows . . . Wrists . . . Hands . . . Upper back . . . Chest and breathing . . . Abdominals . . . Lower back . . . Pelvis . . . Hips . . . Glutes . . . Quads . . . Knees . . . Calves and shins . . . Ankles . . . and finally your feet.

When you've finished scanning your whole body, go back and do one last continuous sweep from head to toe, taking about ten seconds to do it.

When you get skilled at Body Sensing, you become your own best teacher and coach. Once you get used to always using the three steps of Body Sensing, you'll never be left in the dark, wondering what to do next or whether you're doing something right. Remember: 1. Listen carefully. 2. Assess the information. 3. Adjust incrementally.

Breathing: Tapping into Your Chi

Breathing is a skill, just like Body Sensing and focusing. It is at the core of many Eastern disciplines, such as yoga, tantra, chi gung, and meditation. There are books written entirely on the breath and the importance of proper breathing technique. Breathing is one way for chi to enter the body. In yoga, breathing practices are called *prana-*

yama, prana being the equivalent of chi. In running, as in all other types of aerobic exercise, the breath holds the key role of providing oxygen to help fuel active muscles. If you don't get enough oxygen to your muscles, they will be starved of the key component needed for burning fuel. The more efficiently your body can extract oxygen from the air and transfer it to your muscles, the easier your running will feel at any speed. (In Chapter 6, I will give you tips on how to improve your aerobic conditioning and efficiency.)

Many people experience shortness of breath while running. It's not a bad thing. It's *supposed* to happen, especially if you're running faster or farther than your body is conditioned to go. I've had many people admit that they intentionally taught themselves to breathe slowly so no one would know how out of shape they were; meanwhile, they were killing zillions of brain cells to look good. There are also people who experience a large amount of fear when they start to breathe hard. Heavy breathing brings up everyone's worst nightmares and triggers the negative voices of insecurities, such as:

- I'm going to die.
- I can't keep up.
- I can't do this.
- I'm no good.
- This is hard.
- I'm embarrassed.
- I can't believe I'm so out of shape!

Heavy breathing triggers a sense of running out of air, of suffocating, of passing out due to a lack of oxygen or a heart attack.

Below are some causes, and their solutions to why you might breathe more heavily than feels comfortable:

- Low Aerobic Capacity
- Shallow Breathing
- Tension in Your Muscles
- You Just Ate a Huge Dinner

LOW AEROBIC CAPACITY

When you're just starting up a running program, you can expect to be out of breath at first. That's because your muscles are not equipped to take in the additional oxygen supply needed to sustain the increased workload. The best way to increase your aerobic capacity is with LSD. No, it doesn't stand for lysergic acid diethylamide—it stands for long, slow distance running. Doing LSD is what helps increase your aerobic capacity. (I'll cover aerobic training in Chapter 6.) Having a long run in your program ensures that your muscles will be able to keep up with the demand for oxygen. The trick to building aerobic capacity is to do your long run at a conversational pace, meaning that you're moving along at a rate that you never come close to feeling out of breath. You should be able to easily carry on a conversation . . . hopefully with whomever is running with you.

SHALLOW BREATHING

If you're breathing from the upper part of your lungs, you're not getting as much air as you could. A doctor in one of my classes assured me that most of your oxygen exchange happens in the lower lungs. Therefore, if you're breathing into only your upper lungs, you're not getting as much air into your blood supply, even though you might be breathing like a freight train. The cure for this is to breathe deeply, into your lower lungs. If you're short of breath, it's not because you aren't breathing *in* enough—it's because you're not breathing *out* enough. It is important to fully empty your lungs from the bottom so that the used air can be expelled completely, thereby allowing a fresh supply of oxygen back in.

Here's a comparison between what happens when you breathe shallowly and when you belly-breathe. Shallow breathing activates the sympathetic survival instinct—the fight-or-flight response. This, in turn, stimulates stress receptors in the chest and increases your heart rate. The fight-or-flight response triggers the release of the stress hormones cortisol and adrenaline, causing the body to burn blood sugar and store fat. It also raises your blood pressure as a result of the lower oxygenation rate of your muscles, which ultimately overloads the adrenal glands and breaks the body down.

Belly Breathing: The Cure for Shallow Breathing

Belly breathing (diaphragmatic breathing), draws breath into the lower lobes of the lungs, thereby stimulating the body's parasympathetic response. As a result, the body releases a beneficial cocktail of hormones (namely, seretonin and beta-endorphin), lowers heart rate and blood pressure, improves circulation, and produces an overall calming effect and feeling of well-being.

Here's how to belly-breathe. Stand or sit and place your hands over your belly button. Now purse your lips as if you're trying to blow a candle out, and exhale, emptying your lungs by pulling in your belly button toward your spine. When you've blown out as much air as you can, relax your belly, and the inhale will occur naturally. If you want to get additional air into your lungs, you can expand your lower rib cage as you inhale. Practice breathing this way when you're not running, so you can learn the technique without being under physical duress. Once you get comfortable with belly breathing, you can introduce it into your running. Try matching up your breathing with your cadence. I usually breathe out for three steps and breathe in for two, but do what works best for you. It helps if you take more time breathing out than breathing in.

Nose breathing will help you get even more out of your belly breathing. Running regularly for longer distances at a conversational pace is the ideal way to build aerobic capacity. The best way to ensure that you're running at an aerobic pace is to *nose-breathe*. Here's how to do it. The next time you go out for a run, shut your mouth (and keep it shut) and belly-breathe. If you have to open your mouth and gasp for breaths, it means that you're not getting enough oxygen into your lungs, because you're running too fast. Nose breathing is a great self-regulating mechanism because you won't be able to do it if you're either running too fast, not relaxed enough, or inefficient in your movement. When I first started to practice nose breathing I could go for about a minute before I had to breathe through my mouth. As I got more efficient and relaxed with my running form, I was able to nose breathe for longer periods of time. At this point I can do most of my runs without opening my mouth to breathe. It's much more mentally and physically relaxing to run this way.

TENSION IN YOUR MUSCLES

If your muscles are tight or tense, you'll have to breathe harder because it is much more difficult for the oxygenated blood from your lungs to squeeze its way into your muscle cells. It's like the difference between pouring syrup on a pancake and dumping it on a bagel. The bagel is so dense that it won't absorb anything, while the pancakes are more like sponges.

The cure for this is easy. Just relax! Isn't that why you're running to begin with? Don't take yourself so seriously. Drop your shoulders. Smile. Relax your glutes; don't be a tight-ass. Float like a butterfly . . . lighten up!

The biggest help to your breathing will be when you learn to really relax while you're running. Then everything happens more easily. Because you're working more efficiently, your oxygen requirements are lower, and your breathing will take on more of a natural rhythm.

YOU JUST ATE A HUGE DINNER, YOUR 8-YEAR-OLD WANTS TO PLAY TAG, AND YOU FEEL LIKE A BEACHED WHALE

There is no cure for this. Just have fun and do your best to hold on to that dinner.

I've seen runners who have increased their speed and distance simply by learning to improve their breathing. The better you get at identifying your reason for shortness of breath, the sooner you'll be able to do something about it.

Proper breathing is touted as an aid to everything from better vision and brainpower to better sex. There is no end to the value of working with your breath, and with the few suggestions described here, you should be breathing well and easy no matter what your undertaking. Now set this book down in your lap, sit up straight, take a deep breath, and let out a big "ahhhhhhhhhhhhh." See? It's not that hard to breathe well. You just have to remind yourself to do it.

Relaxation: The Path of Least Resistance

I don't know anybody who couldn't stand to have a little more relaxation in his life, me included. But as paradoxical as it sounds, we all have to *work* to make it happen. Interestingly enough, the three best tools to help you learn to relax are Focusing, Body Sensing, and Breathing, which is why Relaxation completes the list of Chi-Skills.

Almost everyone I know lives in some state of density, where there is always a little more going on than we'd like. We all need and crave some spaciousness in our lives, whether it's figurative or literal. I conjure the image of *focused spaciousness* while I'm running. I imagine having openness in my joints and lots of ease in my motion. Nothing feels forced. My movement is free and loose. Now, *that's* the kind of relaxation that I'm talking about.

Master Xu was helping me through yet another T'ai Chi lesson and moving his body without apparently using his muscles. He said to me, "Here, rest your hand on my arm, and keep it there while I go through this movement." I did as he asked.

"Now I'm moving my arm using my muscles," he said, smiling. Indeed he was. I could feel the strength in his forearm. Firm and rigid, it felt like an overdone drumstick at Thanksgiving dinner.

"Now I'm moving with my chi," he said, smiling even more broadly.

Although he was moving his arm in the same motion, the difference was truly dramatic. My closest comparison is the softness I feel in my daughter's arm after she's fallen asleep. Yet there was a distinct feeling of firmness coming from deep within his body, not from his arm. No matter how hard I pushed on his arm, he kept on moving it as if I weren't there. He was able to allow his chi to move me because his muscles were relaxed. Not a lesson goes by in which Master Xu doesn't demonstrate to me the power of relaxation.

A spiritual teacher once gave me a great definition of relaxation. He said, "Relaxation is the absence of unnecessary effort." That sounds simple enough, but it's easier said than done. I began to constantly work with the idea, and when I applied it to my running, it went something like this: the more I could relax my legs and not "effort" with them, the less resistance they created to my forward momentum. The ChiRunning technique allows you to shift the emphasis away from your legs—to get them out of the way so your body can run more easily. It doesn't mean that there's *no* effort, just no *unnecessary* effort. The faster I run, the more I can feel myself move from my center, and the less I need to use my legs. Likewise, the more I gather to my center, the less I use my legs, and the faster I run. The cycle works either way.

Here are some additional benefits to relaxing your muscles. When you are using only your muscles to move your body, you are doing so with a finite amount of energy stored in your muscles. But when you use chi energy to move, you are essentially turning your body into a hybrid machine that operates on two kinds of fuel. It's similar to the hybrid cars that run on gas *and* electricity. The gas engine runs only when necessary (up hills or at higher speeds), and the electric engine takes care of the rest. Similarly, the ChiRunning technique allows you to run with very low muscle usage (gas) because your chi (electricity) is doing most of the work. The better you get at accessing your chi, the less muscle fuel you will consume. It doesn't mean you'll never get tired, but it does mean you'll be moving in such an energy-efficient way that your storehouse of muscular energy will take *much* longer to deplete. Can you imagine what your running would feel like if you ran *mostly* on chi?

I've been using the theme of relaxation to learn to run more effortlessly and also to see how it applies to the rest of my life as well. So far it seems to apply in every situation. As long as I stay relaxed and centered, I more easily accomplish any job set before me—whether it's running a 10K, cooking a meal, or commuting in rush-hour traffic. It seems so much easier to do anything when you offer no resistance to doing it, especially when it's something that you don't like to do! If my legs offer no resistance, the run happens as it should. If I offer no resistance, my life happens as it should.

Running is a place where you can begin to explore the potential freedom of deeply relaxing your body. True Relaxation comes from possessing a strong center and letting go of all else. ChiRunning offers you the tools to have that strong center while relaxing at the same time. It's the principle of Needle in Cotton applied to your running.

Exercise: The 10-Second Relaxation Exercise

This exercise is intended to be done when you're not running, so you can get the feel of it and then transfer it into your running when you need to. (You'll find that you're also developing your Focusing and Body Sensing skills as you practice this exercise.)

Sit in a chair, lie on the floor, or stand upright. Now inhale and try to tense every muscle in your body at the same time. Hold this pose for a count of 10, then let out your breath and release all of the tension you've been holding. Practice this until you feel like you can release every tight muscle in your body. Be very thorough in tensing every muscle, and be equally thorough in relaxing every muscle.

The next step is to do the relaxing part while you're running, and you'll have a great tool to use whenever you need it.

Can you imagine what our world would be like if the four Chi-Skills—Focusing, Body Sensing, Breathing, and Relaxation—were required curricula in all our public schools? These four areas of human experience are, in my mind, such a primary part of our existence that we should all have them as a birthright. We do have these focuses going at different times, but can you imagine having them all engaged at once? The depth of your experience during any activity would be quite different. By practicing these skills in your running, you will eventually find yourself using them in your everyday life, enriching your experience of self and the world around you.

By the way . . . how did you do with holding your posture?

CHAPTER FOUR

Form Focuses:
The Basic Components
of Technique

Spirit needs matter to become substantial; matter needs spirit to become meaningful. —UNKNOWN

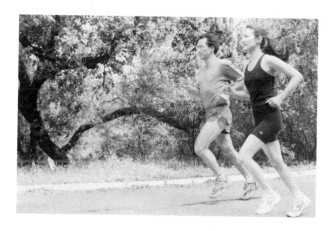

One of our main goals in writing this book was to make your learning process as easy and understandable as possible, so we've divided this chapter into two sections. We'll begin with an overview of the ChiRunning technique so that you know what to expect: how the technique works, what the process will look like along the way, and what the future holds for you as you improve your ChiRunning skills.

In the next section we'll explain all the component parts of the ChiRunning technique, which we call the Form Focuses. It's like a list of job descriptions for all the parts of your body that will be involved in your running.

Part I: An Overview of the ChiRunning Form: A Revolutionary Approach to Effortless, Injury-Free Running

We just want you to have an overview of what you'll be working toward—a carrot to keep you on the path to learning good running form.

When ChiRunning is more fully incorporated into your running, there is a wonderful opportunity to experience the effortless aspect of the running mentioned in the subtitle of this book. Learning ChiRunning is not effortless. We know that. But as more aspects of this form become incorporated into your running, there will be times when you may experience that delightful feeling of "I could run forever." I experience truly effortlessness running about 60% of the time. The other 40% of the time I am working toward those moments of bliss. I am always making corrections, trying something new, practicing, and focusing on my weak areas. I love that part too, but when I do drop into "the zone" it is pure delight.

Many of our clients have sent letters chronicling that effortless experience you'll be working toward. Jeanne wrote, "Danny, I just have to say it again . . . ChiRunning rocks! Seriously, this morning it was like I had no legs running—I was just floating! Love it! Thanks!"

Consider this chapter a complete and detailed reference of all the ChiRunning focuses, but be aware that it is not presented in the sequence in which you should learn the technique. We will give you the best sequence of learning these focuses in Chapter 5, where we get you started with ten specific lessons. After successfully teaching thousands of runners ChiRunning, the sequence of these lessons has proven to be the quickest and easiest way to learn the technique.

The Form Focuses fall into six categories: posture, lean, lower body, pelvic rotation, upper body, and the triad of cadence, gears and stride length. In this chapter we explain the logic and the how-to of each Form Focus. Since all of the details about every Form Focus are in this chapter, you will be referred back to this chapter extensively in Chapter 5 and throughout the rest of the book. It's a good idea to add plastic note tabs to mark each of the Form Focus areas for instant access anytime you have questions about a particular aspect of the technique.

As you read this chapter, just take in the information . . . and relax. You don't need to learn it all right away and there will be no pop quizzes.

THE SIX FORM FOCUS GROUPS

Posture

The most basic concept behind ChiRunning and the way it optimally works is that you create a straight line with your posture, from the crown of your head to the bottoms of your feet. We call this your *Column*. When your Column is aligned properly, your body weight is supported primarily by your structure, not your muscles.

Lean

The idea with ChiRunning is to allow your Column to fall gently forward in a controlled way, allowing gravity to pull you forward. As you fall forward, the rearward force of the road pulls your support leg out behind you, allowing your leading foot to land underneath your center of mass, catching you from falling. You then land on that leg, momentarily supporting your weight as your Column passes over it. The foot gently lands, with a midfoot strike at the bottom of your Column (never in front of it) and the force of the road then pulls that support leg out behind you.

Lower Body

As you fall forward, you gently peel your feet off the ground to keep up with your fall. You do not use your legs for propulsion in any way. You don't push off with your quads, calves, or toes and you don't pull with your hamstrings. We call it the "passive lower leg" because your legs are used only for support between strides and nothing else.

Pelvic Rotation

The movement of your legs creates a counter-rotation between your upper body and your lower body, and your pelvis (if allowed) rotates around its central axis (along the spine). If your pelvis does not rotate, you'll absorb the force of the road with your knees, quads, hips, or lower back. Allowing your pelvis to rotate allows you to cooperate with the force of the road coming at you, without your body absorbing any of it.

Upper Body

In ChiRunning your upper body is leading the show. One of our instructors says, "Run with your heart first." In this way you're cooperating with the pull of gravity as you allow yourself to fall forward. The counter-balance to your upper body falling forward is your elbows swinging to the rear.

Cadence, Stride Length, and Gears

The next part of the technique that you'll learn is cadence, gears, and stride length. In ChiRunning there's one thing that never changes: your cadence. That's the rate at which your feet strike the ground, measured in strides per minute. One thing in ChiRunning that *does* constantly change is your stride length. It's simple: as your speed increases, so does the length of your stride. Likewise, as you slow down, your stride shortens proportionately. Having your stride length change relative to the speed you're running equates to the gears in a car or a bicycle.

With ChiRunning, your recommended cadence will probably be quicker than you are used to at first. You'll also notice that at slower speeds, your stride length will be shorter than you're used to. You can watch a very clear example of this on the ChiRunning DVD. I run in four different speeds, all with the same cadence, but you'll clearly see the difference in stride lengths with each successive gear.

ADVANCED STAGES OF EFFORTLESS RUNNING
The Increased Use of Core Strength

As you get into more advanced stages, you'll learn that your core strength is what helps keep you balanced in your forward fall. You'll learn to play with this balance to increase or reduce speed, to go up or down hills, to help recover from fatigue, and to have fun. As your core gets stronger, you'll be able to run faster or longer without significantly increasing your effort level.

Use of the Ligaments and Tendons

The ChiRunning technique creates a counter-rotation between your hips and shoulders, causing your spine to gently twist. This twisting motion pulls on the ligaments and tendons in your shoulders, spine, and hips, which in turn act like rubber bands wanting to return your spinal twist to its neutral position. With this rubber-band effect, your arms and legs are moving because of the stretch and recoil of your ligaments and tendons, *not* the contraction of your muscles. This nonmuscular action results in an incredibly energy-efficient running technique. Your ligaments and tendons do not burn fuel (which requires oxygen and glycogen), so less lactic acid is produced when you run. Since your muscles are not being broken down, there is less recovery time needed. And as you run, your muscles learn to relax and let go of tension while your tendons become more flexible and resilient. As gravity pulls you forward, your body moves *in response to* your forward fall. Once you are skilled in the basic Form Focuses you'll be able to employ these advanced techniques.

I'm sure this sounds like an awful lot to think about and do while you're running. That's why we recommend that you practice your ChiRunning technique one focus at a time. You have plenty of time to incorporate it into your running, so don't feel rushed. You will get specific instructions on all of this in the next section.

Although we've done our best in this book to illustrate what the ChiRunning form looks like, it helps tremendously to watch the ChiRunning DVD or to get personal instruction from a Certified ChiRunning Instructor. In our recent survey the number one concern people had was that they were not sure if they were doing it right. Having an instructor watch you is very helpful, and the DVD gives you a visual experience that we cannot get across in a book. Learning ChiRunning with a friend is another good option.

PART II: THE FORM FOCUSES

The aim of ChiRunning is to convert running from a sport to a *practice*. When you take on something as a *practice*, you approach it with the mind-set of improving either your skill or yourself. Either way, the nature of a practice done well is to leave you with more than when you started. When you practice something, you transform it into being process-oriented rather than goal-oriented. With ChiRunning, what you are practicing are the Form Focuses.

The ChiRunning principle that best represents the Form Focuses is Needle in Cotton, or *alignment and relaxation*. Every Form Focus is designed to address either energy efficiency or injury prevention by either aligning or relaxing some part of your body. Energy efficiency and injury prevention are two topics you should always have in the back of your mind when running. The beauty of the ChiRunning focuses is that you can practice most of them all day long, not just while you're running. Good posture, relaxed muscles, and great breathing can and should be a part of your everyday life.

Here, again, are the six groups of Form Focuses.

1. Posture
2. Lean
3. Lower body
4. Pelvic rotation
5. Upper body
6. Gears, cadence, and stride length

POSTURE

Good, efficient running technique is based on alignment and relaxation. So let's begin with alignment. The Basic Rule of Alignment is this: Whenever you're running, you should have as many of your body parts as possible moving in the same direction you're headed.

It's a very simple rule, but you'd be surprised by how many people I see breaking this rule. Here are some examples. If your arms are swinging side to side when you're running, you're wasting your energy. If you're bouncing up and down when you run, you're not totally moving in the direction you're headed. If your shoulders sway from side to side when you run, like Rocky Balboa, you're moving inefficiently. And this is the short list! If any part of your body is not moving generally in the same direction you're heading, not only is it *not* helping you, but you could be wearing out your joints because they're moving in a way that they weren't designed to move. It all comes down to getting aligned with the direction you're headed.

Here are the six sequential steps to get your posture aligned:

1. Align your feet and legs
2. Align your upper body by lengthening your spine
3. Level your pelvis and engage your core
4. Create your column
5. The one-legged posture stance
6. The "C" Shape

We'll begin with your postural alignment because having good posture is the cornerstone of the ChiRunning technique and crucial to building strong core muscles. When your posture is correct, energy or chi flows through your body unhindered, in much the same way that water flows through a straight pipe more easily than a bent one. Running with your posture out of alignment can create tension, fatigue, discomfort, and even pain. When your posture is aligned properly, your *structure* is supporting the weight of your body instead of your muscles.

The principle of Needle in Cotton also applies to posture. When your posture is correctly aligned, you have a centerline or axis that runs the length of your body. When that centerline is straight and strong, it is the "needle" that supports your body, which then allows your arms and legs to relax and become like "cotton."

Many people tend to think that posture applies mostly to their trunk. When asked to stand up straight, they don't think about what their legs are doing—they simply adjust their *upper body*. But your *lower body* is equally important, especially if you're a runner. So let's begin with aligning your feet and legs, since they are used during the support phase of your stride.

Posture: 1. Aligning Your Feet and Legs

Here's what can happen if your feet splay out when you run. Landing with your feet pointing out makes it more likely that you will strike the ground with the outside edge of your heel. This will weaken the medial ligaments and tendons of your ankle, because you're rolling diagonally across your foot onto your big toe, which can cause you to overpronate. As you swing through your stride, this motion creates a twist in your lower leg, which in turn puts stress on the medial meniscus tendon in your knee. This is a big cause of runner's knee as well as iliotibial band and hip injuries. Read more about knee issues in chapter 9, page 230.

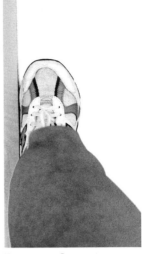

Figure 9—Correct
knee/foot alignment

1. Align your feet so that they are pointed in the direction you're headed, parallel and hip width apart. To get your feet aligned, don't just point your feet forward; rotate each leg medially until your foot points forward. With each step you'll be building stronger adductor muscles, and eventually your feet won't turn out while running. When that time comes, all overpronation-related injuries could become a thing of the past.

2. Next, balance the pressure on the bottoms of your feet. Make sure

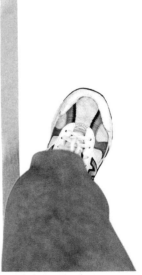

Figure 10—Incorrect
knee/foot alignment

your weight is distributed evenly between your left foot and your right foot. Then balance your feet so you feel even pressure between the heels and the balls of your feet. Finally, balance your feet so that there is equal pressure between the lateral (outside) side of your feet, and your arches. Find this "sweet spot" and relax your feet. Make sure you are not gripping with your toes. Keeping your feet relaxed and soft throughout your stride is key to learning how to run with passive lower legs.

Injury Prevention Tip: After aligning your legs and feet, soften your knees so they're not locked. Locking your knees puts a lot of stress on your kneecaps and can lead to knee injuries.

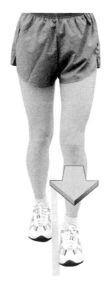

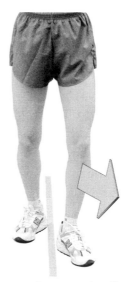

Figure 11—Correct leg/foot alignment

Figure 12—Incorrect leg/foot alignment

Learning Tip: To keep your feet pointing forward while you're running, pretend you have a stripe painted on the ground and your feet are lined up on either side of the stripe.

Injury Prevention Tip: I was an overpronator and had chronic knee pain whenever I hit the 20-mile mark. I cured it by practicing these simple focuses on a daily basis. When I'm tired, though, I still need to remind myself to rotate my knee in when walking or running. If your feet naturally splay out quite a bit, it might feel uncomfortable at first to point them forward. If this is the case, just back off of your rotation until the discomfort *almost* disappears, and your feet are still pointing more forward than they normally do. It may take several months, or longer, for you to get your feet pointing forward. However if you work at it gradually, you can make this correction without injury.

Posture: 2. Align Your Upper Body by Lengthening Your Spine

Now that we have the legs and feet aligned, let's move to the upper body. Here is how to align your spine in three easy steps:

1. Spread apart the middle finger and the thumb of one hand and place them just under your collarbone, with your palm resting on your chest. Place the thumb of your other hand in your belly button with your fingers resting over your lower abs.
2. Now lift with your upper hand (using your collarbone like a handle) while pulling down with your lower hand. This motion will straighten your upper spine, which increases your lung capacity. As you do this, soften your shoulders and don't arch your lower back or stick your chest out. Just envision lengthening your spine and creating space between each vertebrae (figure 13).
3. To align your head and neck, remove your hand from your upper chest and place it on the back of your neck at the base of the skull. Now brush your neck in an upward direction or lift the base of the skull while lengthening the back side of your neck. This will allow your chin to drop naturally. One way to accomplish all three steps in one simple motion is to just lengthen the back of your neck and you'll see how it lengthens your entire spine (figure 14).

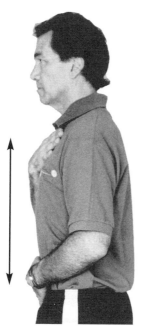
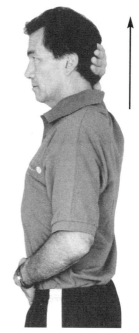

Figure 13—Hands aligning upper body

Figure 14—Lengthen back of neck with hand

Lifting up on the back of the neck will lighten your step and create a force in the opposite direction to coming down onto your feet (figure 15).

Regularly remembering to lengthen the back of your neck will ensure that your posture line stays long and straight. The feeling that you should have is that your spine is lengthening, from your tailbone to the crown of your skull. It's like someone is lifting you by pulling up from the crown of your head. This is a great focus to practice all day long whether you're standing, driving your car, or sitting at your desk.

As you do this upper body alignment, be sure to soften your knees; don't lock them. Lengthening your spine opens your chest and allows you to breathe more fully. Running with your upper body hunched over can reduce your oxygen intake by up to 30%.

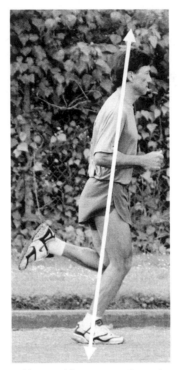

Figure 15—Upward force counteracts gravity

Posture: 3. Level Your Pelvis and Engage Your Core

Here's a way to get your core muscles engaged in your running. It's called leveling your pelvis, and it is a key component to maintaining good posture while running.

There are many reasons for engaging your core muscles in this way. The three primary reasons are:

1. To maintain a straight Column while running (or walking)
2. To stabilize the pelvis during movement
3. To create a more powerful connection between the pelvis and legs, unifying the movement of the whole lower body

In this section, we are going to focus on the first reason. When we get to pelvic rotation, we will thoroughly explain the second and third reasons.

Creating and maintaining a straight Column while running is the cornerstone of ChiRunning and a crucial component for energy efficiency and injury prevention.

Master Xu uses the metaphor of the pelvis being like a bowl. If it's tipped forward, it will spill its contents. Whereas, if it's level, it can hold the contents without spilling (see figure 16). If the contents of the bowl represent your chi, then as you tip your pelvis, you "spill your chi" (see figure 17). Keeping your pelvis level does two things: it strengthens your core muscles (lower abdominals), allowing you to hold your Column straight when running, and it brings your focus to your center, where your true power lies, allowing you to "contain" your chi. This also allows you to feel physically and energetically centered in your movement.

Exercise: Leveling Your Pelvis

Here's how to level your pelvis:

1. To feel your lower abdominals, put your thumb in your belly button with the rest of your fingers spread beneath your thumb and resting on your lower abs. To feel your lower abs working, do a fake cough and you'll feel them contracting.

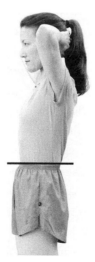 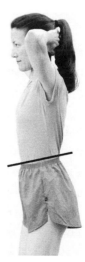

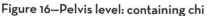

Figure 16—Pelvis level: containing chi   Figure 17—Pelvis tilted: spilling chi

2. To level your pelvis, contract those lower abs by lifting up on the front side of your pelvis.
3. Don't clench your glutes while doing this exercise. Just isolate and work your lower abs. It should feel like you're doing a crunch except that you're standing up. I call it the Vertical Crunch.
4. Each time you lift up on the front of your pelvis, hold it for ten seconds and then relax.

Injury Prevention Tip: If your bowl is tipped (anterior pelvic tilt), much of your core strength will be unavailable to you because your core muscles will remain unused or underdeveloped. In order to avoid tipping your bowl, you'll need to strengthen your abs while at the same time relaxing your lower back muscles. Too much curvature in your lower back means that your abdominal muscles are overextended and your lower back muscles are too contracted. *Some* curve in your lower back is healthy. Too much curvature can compress the discs in your spine and create pressure on your spinal cord. This can seriously cramp your style. I've been there. As you create more of a balance between the front and back sides of your body, there will be more spaciousness throughout your vertebrae and much less chance for lower back pain or injury.

Practice this exercise when you are not moving, so you can get a sense of how it feels, then bring that feeling into your movement. Do this exercise anytime, whenever you find yourself standing in line, when you're carrying groceries, and especially when you've got a kid on your shoulders. As your lower abs get stronger you will then be able to do it correctly during your running.

Leveling your pelvis is a great exercise for those of you with lower back problems because it strengthens your abs while relaxing your back muscles. The more often you remember to do it, the sooner your lower abdominal muscles will get strong enough to hold your pelvis level as you run.

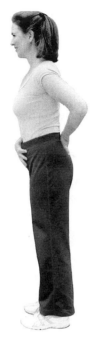
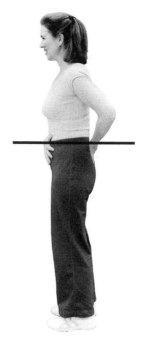

Figure 18—Core muscles not engaged

Figure 19—Core muscles engaged, pelvis level

Injury Prevention Tip. You want to create a level pelvis but you don't want to go past level and create a posterior pelvic tilt. This will cause too much tension and will most likely engage the glutes and restrict your leg swing. You want to be strong, not tense. I have rarely seen anyone who has a natural posterior pelvic tilt. The key to leveling our pelvis is to isolate your lower abs and use only them.

Exercise: Strengthen Your Abs

This is an alternative exercise that will help you to strengthen your abdominal muscles and tilt your pelvis without engaging your glutes. It is particularly good if you have too much curvature in your lumbar spine.

1. Lie on your back with your knees bent and your heels touching your butt.
2. Gently press your lower back into the floor so that there is no gap between your spine and the floor.
3. Now, let your legs slowly straighten as your feet walk away from your lower back. Walk *only as far as you can* without letting your lower back lose contact with the floor. When your lower back starts to pull up from the floor, stop and hold the position for thirty seconds, then walk back up to your starting position. It does not matter how far you go before your back comes up. Remember, Gradual Progress. This exercise will strengthen your lower abs—without engaging your glutes—and give you a distinct feeling of holding your pelvis up in front while lying in a supine position. Repeat this exercise five times and hold your spine against the floor for thirty seconds each time.

Exercise: Strengthen Your Core

Here's a second exercise to help strengthen the core muscles that stabilize your pelvis. There are two versions depending on how strong your core is to begin with.

Beginning version: Lie on your back with your knees bent and your feet flat on the ground. Keeping your shoulders on the floor, raise your butt off the floor and make a "plank" with your body so you have a straight line running from your shoulders to your knees. Hold this position for twenty seconds. Then lower your body back down to the floor and rest for a few seconds. Repeat this exercise five times. Add one repeat each week until you get up to ten repeats and feel comfortable doing them all. Then graduate to the next version.

Advanced version: Sit on the floor, legs parallel and straight out in front of you with your upper body upright. Place your palms on the floor right next to your hips, with your fingers pointing forward and your elbows locked. Keeping your feet where they are, lift up your pelvis until your body makes a horizontal "plank" supported by your lower legs and your arms. Hold this position for twenty seconds, then lower your body back down to the floor. Repeat this five times and add one repeat each week until you get up to ten repeats.

If you want an advanced version of the advanced version, go into the horizontal plank position and straighten one of your legs so you have a straight line running horizontally from the top of your head to the bottom of your foot. Hold it there for twenty seconds and repeat by straightening the opposite leg. Alternate legs for however many repeats you can stand it. If you're still not challenged enough, have a friend sit on your stomach while you're in the plank position. This will be a true test of the strength of—you guessed it—your ego.

> **Injury Prevention Tip.** Stand with your feet together and don't level your pelvis. Shift your weight from one leg to the other. You will notice that your hips move side to side. Now, level your pelvis and hold it level as you shift your weight from one leg to the other. You will notice that your hips don't go side to side. The side-to-side movement of the hips, due to disengaged core muscles, is the number one cause of hip bursitis and iliotibial band syndrome. The side-to-side motion of the hips is more common in women than in men.

Posture: 4. Create Your Column

I would say that 80% of all the runners I teach start off by standing with their hips too far forward and their legs sloped to the rear, their shoulders back, and their knees locked.

If you stand with your hips forward, over the years you'll begin to feel compression in your lower back. This could eventually lead to either a compressed disc in your spine, tight neck muscles, or hip bursitis. Needless to say, it's not a great way to stand . . . and it's even a worse way to run. Leading with your hips while running can magnify the compressive force to your lower back, and believe me, you don't want to go there.

The following exercise will bring your hips into alignment with your shoulders, allowing your upper body to balance directly over your hips. Your shoulders, hips, and ankles will now create your Column (see figure 21). When your Column is aligned, your body weight will be supported by your structure, allowing your muscles to do what they're supposed to be doing whenever you're ChiRunning . . . resting and relaxing.

Exercise: Create Your Column
This exercise is best done standing sideways in front of a full-length mirror. It is most effective to do this with a friend or in a ChiRunning workshop with a Certified ChiRunning Instructor.

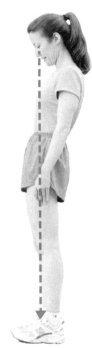

1. Align your legs and feet, lengthen your spine, and level your pelvis as above.
2. Now, without moving your body drop your chin and look down to see if you can see your feet. If you can see your shoelaces, it's a good bet that your dots are connected and your Column is in a straight line.
3. If you *can't* see your shoelaces, it means that your hips are too far forward. Correct this by placing your fingertips on your hip bones and pushing your hips to the rear while keeping your shoulders directly over your feet. (Of course, if you can't see your shoelaces for anatomical reasons, such as a large chest or a protruding stomach because you're pregnant or overweight, have no fear. Just use the mirror and look at a side view of your body.)

Figure 20—Common posture today: incorrect—hips forward

4. Once you can see your shoelaces, slowly lift your head up to where your eyes are looking straight ahead. Don't move the rest of your body—just lift your head. Now, look at yourself in the mirror. Are your shoulders, hip bones, and ankles in a straight line? If they are, that's great.
5. Once again, soften your knees and balance the pressure on your feet, front to back and side to side.
6. When your dots are connected, Body Sense and take a "physical

snapshot" of what it feels like to stand this way. Memorize that feeling so you can remember it whenever you're standing around.

If you're used to standing with your abdominals relaxed and your hips forward, this adjustment might make you feel like you're bent at the waist with your butt sticking out. Just ask a friend to take a look at you or look in a mirror to see if you are bent over. They'll probably tell you that you're straight as an arrow, but it'll *feel* like you're bent forward at the waist. The easiest way to check if you're off balance in any way is to refer back to the bottoms of your feet. Are they still balanced

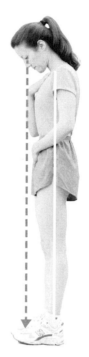

Figure 21—Correct posture—hips aligned

front/back, side to side and lateral/medial? They should be.

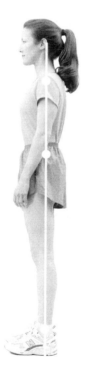

Figure 22—Proper alignment of shoulder, hip, and ankle

Here's a fun test to see if your dots are connected.

Stand in a relaxed position and ask a friend to gently pull down on your shoulders (from behind). If you're slouching and your dots aren't lined up, your hips will move forward when your friend pulls down on your shoulders.

Next, stand with your feet and legs aligned, your upper body tall and straight, and your dots connected, meaning that your hips are slightly back and your shoulders are slightly

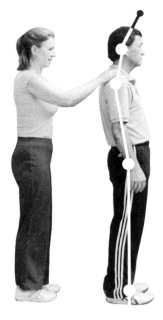
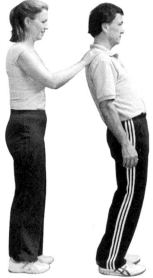
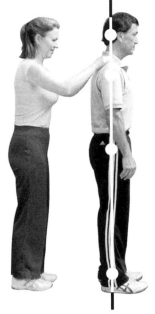

Figure 23—Stand with your core relaxed

Figure 24—Pull down gently on the shoulders (notice the hips move forward)

Figure 25—Pull down with your core engaged

forward. When you're all lined up, have your friend pull down on your shoulders. You will feel a remarkable difference. This is a major "aha" moment in all my workshops.

Posture: 5. The One-Legged Posture Stance

The one-legged posture stance will train your core muscles to hold your posture straight during the support phase of your stride. When you are running you are moving in a series of one-legged posture stances. As you will see when we talk about lower body focuses, you do not push off or pull with your legs. They are there for support only. This is the primary job your legs do in ChiRunning, so it is important to get a clear Body Sense of the one-legged posture stance when done correctly.

Exercise: One-Legged Posture Stance

1. Create your Column.
2. Once you feel you've got the sensation of good posture in your body, stand with your feet *together* and maintain your Column while alternately supporting your weight on one leg, and then the other. Simply lift one heel off the ground so that your weight shifts onto one leg. Hold this for five seconds and then switch legs and support yourself with your other leg. Always keep your knees slightly bent.
3. Feel each foot down at the bottom of your one-legged posture stance with your entire Column balanced directly over it. Memorize this feeling in your body. This is the one-legged posture stance.

Note: The one-legged posture stance will also be referred to as the support phase of your stride.

Posture: 6. The "C" Shape

Now that you know how to align your posture and feel your Column, here's an exercise designed to get it all to happen in a split second while you're running. It's quicker and easier than trying to go through all the various steps while you're cruising down the road.

Exercise: The "C" Shape

1. Stand with your arms at your sides, your legs aligned, your pelvis dropped in front (not level), and your chin slightly up, as it probably usually is.
2. Now, in one gentle motion, level your pelvis and lengthen the back of your neck. If you trace a line from your chin up and over the top of your head, down your back, under the pelvis, and up to your pubic bone it looks like a "C" shape. Your chin is the beginning of the "C" shape, while your pubic bone is the other end of the "C." Do this *slowly* five times, starting each time with your pelvis dropped in front and your chin up, and ending with your pelvis level and the back of your neck lengthened.

3. Now, count to three, and when you say "three," lengthen the back of your neck and level your pelvis in one swift full-body motion. One . . . two . . . three—"C" shape! Practice standing in place and putting yourself into the "C" shape in one swift motion a few times. Try it at a very relaxed running pace and get used to doing it while you're moving. You'll definitely notice a difference in the solidity of your body as you run.

As you can see, there's a *lot* to posture. When I teach all-day classes, we spend at least one third of the class practicing posture. But nobody complains when they see how much easier it makes their running. The better your posture is, the less you have to worry about hurting your body or overworking your legs. It's as simple as that.

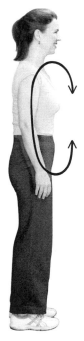
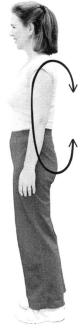

Figure 26—Correct posture showing the "C" shape

Figure 27—Incorrect posture

THE LEAN: GRAVITY-ASSISTED RUNNING

I use the word *lean* to get runners to engage the assistance of gravity by falling forward with the full length of their body. When you think of leaning, think of your entire Column leaning as a unit. If your Column is not straight, gravity pulls on the bent, misaligned parts in ways that can inhibit the gentle forward fall and cause more stress.

As we've discussed, leaning puts gravity in your favor because you are falling forward instead of your legs having to *push* you, which we all know can be tiring. When you are standing upright, gravity is pulling straight down on your body along your centerline. As soon as you allow your body to fall forward, your center of mass moves in front of your point of contact with the ground. Gravity will then pull downward on your center of mass, making you fall forward, with your ankles acting like "hinges" as your body tips forward. Your job then, is to learn to balance yourself in a *very* slight forward lean so you're always falling, but not on your face. I love having gravity do the work.

Your lean is your "gas pedal." If you want to go faster, you lean slightly more, in very small increments, and if you want to run slowly, you lean less. As you *increase* your lean, your *abdominals* work to keep your Column straight while you're falling forward. An increase in lean allows gravity to pull you forward at a faster rate, and voilà— your speed is no longer dictated by your leg strength but rather is controlled by your ability to relax your lower body (which we'll talk about later in this section).

Exercise: Learning How to Lean
This exercise will teach you how to lean forward from your ankles, instead of bending at the waist.

1. Find a rigid support at least waist high—a wall in your home, a tree, a fence, a car.
2. Stand facing the support with your toes one shoe length away from the bottom of the wall, which is pretty close. Pay very close attention to keeping your posture aligned *at all times* by engaging your "C" shape, and keep the pressure on the bottom of your feet *evenly*

balanced throughout the entire exercise. Bend your elbows with your hands out in front of you a couple of inches from the support.

3. Now, without looking down, drop your mental attention down to the bottoms of your feet. Then simply relax your lower legs and you'll fall forward, catching your fall with your hands as they come into contact with the support. When you fall forward, be sure to keep your Column straight and your ankles relaxed.

If you're truly relaxing your ankles, your heels won't come up off the ground as your body falls forward. If you're doing it right, you won't feel any increase in pressure under the balls of your feet as you lean forward. If you do feel an increase in pressure under the balls of your feet, it means that your calves and shins are tensing instead of relaxing. Practice the leaning exercise until you can feel your ankles, feet, and lower legs completely relax whenever you're leaning.

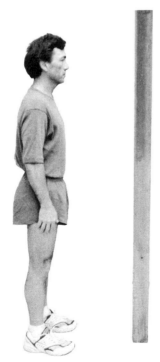 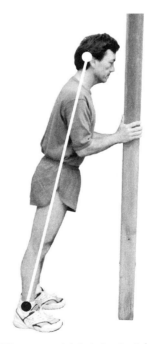

Figure 28—Begin with your posture stance

Figure 29—Maintain straight posture while leaning

Bending at the waist overworks your lower back muscles (see figure 30).

Also, don't pull your head up when you lean or you will throw your posture out of alignment (see figure 31).

4. After you fall against the support and catch yourself, push yourself back upright and repeat this exercise until you have a good Body Sense of leaning. Keep your heels down, Column straight, pelvis level, ankles and calves relaxed.

In summary, the three steps you should use *every time* you engage your lean are:

1. Check in with your posture line.
2. Drop your attention to the bottoms of your feet and keep your feet hitting where they are.
3. Let your Column fall in front of where your feet are hitting.

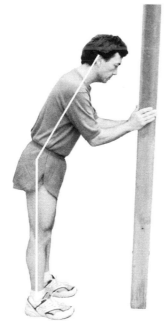 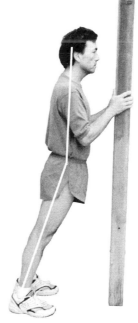

Figure 30—Don't bend at the waist

Figure 31—Posture bent the wrong way: weak abdominals

Exercise: The Window of Lean

You can most definitely lean too much. One of the biggest mistakes of those learning ChiRunning is to use too much lean at first. The trick is to learn to balance yourself in your forward lean. How do you tell if you're leaning too much or not enough? Here's how. I call it the "window of lean."

If you feel your calves or shins getting tight or sore, you are probably leaning too much. Your lower leg muscles are working to keep you from falling on your face. If you run too upright, your legs have to push you forward. When you're in the "window," you feel little if any tension anywhere in your legs because you're leaning in a balanced state . . . not too far forward and not too upright.

Try this:

1. Run upright for a few seconds, balancing yourself directly over your feet, and Body Sense your legs pushing you forward.
2. Add 1 inch of lean to your Column (That's not very much . . . miniscule, in fact.) and run for ten more seconds.
3. Now, exaggerate your lean until you feel your lower legs begin to work to keep you from falling too far forward.
4. Back off of your exaggerated lean until the tension in your lower legs goes away and you find that sweet spot of perfect balance.
5. Back off the lean even more and notice how your body slows down.

Practice these steps to perfect your lean. Then, as you develop your running program, you'll be adding or subtracting small increments of lean to increase or decrease your speed without overworking your legs.

> **Visualization:** One of my favorite examples is the Road Runner of cartoon fame. He has a great lean while his feet are spinning like a wheel behind him.

Exercise: Build Abdominal Strength Without Moving a Muscle

Here's an exercise for those of you who want additional practice leaning and who want to build lower abdominal muscles when you're not running.

Find a table or a stationary object where you can lean against your upper quads while letting your body fall forward. Hold yourself in a straight line while maintaining a lean and you'll get a great abdominal workout without moving a muscle. When you do supplemental strength training, it's always best to build your muscles in the motion in which they will be used. This exercise trains your abdominal muscles to hold your posture straight while leaning forward at the same time.

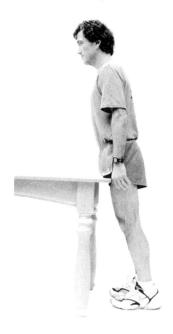

Figure 32—Lean against a table, keeping your posture straight

Exercise: Using Your Y'chi

Y'chi is all about combining your knowledge of what needs to happen with your intention and using your eyes to direct all that energy in the direction your body's heading (see page 44). To add even more power to this, visualize your body filled with energy coursing through every part of it. Then gather all that energy along with your own intent, direct it out through your eyes, and send it forward to a point or object in the distance, *without ever breaking your visual connection.*

Here's an exercise to help you learn to apply y'chi to your running and get a good feel for leaning. You can use this to run or walk more effortlessly and efficiently.

1. The next time you're out running or walking, focus your eyes on a distant object or spot on the horizon and then run or walk toward that object *without ever breaking your gaze.* If you're on a curvy

trail, just choose a point you can focus on until you have to make a turn.

2. Focus on that spot intensely, with your eyes. Don't break visual connection.

3. If you are in the early stages of practicing ChiRunning, keep in mind your good posture and leveling your pelvis. But as you master the technique, you'll want to Body Sense your whole body being aligned and all of that focused energy coming out of your eyes toward your goal. Although you are leaning forward, your y'chi will help you naturally fall into greater alignment while you're leaning. Your whole body will follow the direction of your eyes.

4. Feel yourself being pulled forward by your y'chi, like a giant bungee cord. Think of Spider-Man shooting a strand of web out from his hand. He sends it out to stick to the building in front of him and then allows the strand to pull him forward through the air. It's a neat trick, but you can do the same thing with your *eyes* . . . and without having to wear a silly costume.

The bottom line, though, is that your eyes are directing the movement. Y'chi is the ability to direct your chi toward a visual "goal" through the use of your eyes.

Lower Body Form Focuses

Now we get to the question of what your legs do while running. The answer is, as little as possible. The hardest part in learning the ChiRunning technique may be learning to *not* use your legs. It is well worth the effort to learn to relax this part of your body. In doing so you will reduce the majority of running injuries. Here's an overview:

- The passive lower leg
- Swing your legs to the rear
- The midfoot strike

THE PASSIVE LOWER LEG

This might sound completely counterintuitive, but the faster I run, the less I "use" my legs. This follows the principle of Needle in Cotton because the more I lean my Column (the "needle") into the pull of gravity, the more I need to relax and make "cotton" out of my arms and legs.

We call it the passive lower leg. We are all so used to using our legs for propulsion in running that to take some of that emphasis away represents a shift in dependence from a familiar muscle group (the legs) to a less familiar group (the abdominals).

Exercise: Pick Up Your Heels

In ChiRunning, you won't be pushing yourself forward with each stride. In fact, all you have to do is pick up your feet to keep up with your forward fall. In terms of energy efficiency, it takes much less energy to pick up your feet than it does to push your body forward. The best way to pick up your feet is to focus on lifting your heel.

To feel the difference between lifting up your heel and pushing off with your feet, try these two drills:

1. First, stand in place in your best posture.
2. Peel your foot off the ground, heel first, like a stamp off a new roll. An easy way to peel your foot off the ground is to just think of *lifting up your ankle* and making your foot floppy. Do this several times on each foot to get the feel.
3. Now, walk in place this way for a while, peeling your feet and relaxing your ankles.

Then try this:

1. Run in place for five seconds.
2. Now peel your feet up for five seconds.
3. Run in place again for five seconds.
4. Peel up your feet again for five seconds.

All done? Now I'm going to give you a choice: you can do one or the other for *three hours*. Which one would expend less energy? If you chose peeling your feet up, you get a gold star. If you chose running in place for three hours, you get a case of shin splints.

> **Injury Prevention Tip:** Pushing off with your toes creates too much up-and-down motion and overworks your lower legs. Picking up your feet allows your body to run smoothly along the ground without bouncing. This will ensure that you're moving horizontally toward your goal, instead of bouncing along like a rabbit, fighting gravity with each step.

When you pick up your feet, you'll avoid many common injuries, including shin splints, calf pulls, Achilles tendonitis, plantar fasciitis, and knee injuries. You'll also avoid everyone's most feared accident: tripping and falling.

Exercise: Walk with Peeling Up the Foot

Now you're going to practice lifting up your foot while walking.

1. Rather than practicing it while walking in place, walk around. As you do, focus on peeling your foot off the ground and lifting your heel over the ankle of the other foot.
2. Focus on just lifting the ankle and letting the foot dangle. This will make you take smaller strides, which is a good thing. Concentrate on peeling the foot off the ground and letting the ankle float up behind you in a smooth circular movement. Don't be concerned with lifting your entire foot over the opposite ankle . . . just lift your heel up and over your opposite ankle.
3. Every now and then, walk your normal way so that you can become totally familiar with the difference between pushing off and picking up.

When you walk in the conventional way you can feel every muscle and tendon in your lower legs working. When you switch to peeling your feet off the ground, all of that muscle work and tension will disappear and your lower legs will remain completely relaxed no matter how far or fast you walk.

Devote every day to walking this way. Practice it all the time. This is how you want to walk or run through life. If you practice peeling up your feet, your motion will be smoother along the ground and create less impact. Bring Body Sensing into your running. It seems so simple, yet is so important—and it's crucial to staving off lower leg injuries.

Exercise: The Sand Pit Exercise

If you feel you're having a hard time learning to pick up your feet while running, this is a great exercise. It's actually one of my favorite exercises, and one that I give to all the beginning classes. It's a fun way to learn how to do something very different than you're used to. If you're one of those runners who has a hard time breaking yourself of the habit of over-using your lower legs, you'll learn how to not push off with your feet. Many runners have had remarkable results with this exercise after doing it for only five minutes! Practice this all the time when you're running or walking. It's also a great way to learn how to run in the sand or snow.

1. Find a place to run in the sand. If you live near a beach, this is relatively easy. If you live inland, it's more difficult but not impossible. Go to your local high school track and see if there's a broad-jump pit somewhere. There usually is.
2. Level a path in the sand so you can easily see your footprints.
3. Walk across the sand peeling your feet up with each step. Your goal is to leave clean, undisturbed footprints in the sand. If there is a little crater at the front of each footprint it means that you are either pushing off with your toes with each step or holding some amount of tension in your ankles. Keep trying until you can make perfect imprints with the soles of your shoes every time.
4. Next, level a clean path in the sand and this time run across the sand with a short stride, picking up your feet as you go. Then go back and look at your tracks. If there's a little crater at the front of

each footprint, it means that you are either pushing off with your toes or holding tension in your ankles.

5. Again, make a clean path across the sand, except this time really focus on keeping your lower legs totally limp as you run, and peeling your feet up off the sand with each step. Have the image in mind that you don't want to disturb the sand as you run across it.

6. Continue to run across the sand as many times as you need in order to leave footprints that are clean and undisturbed. This exercise forces you to relax all the muscles in your lower legs, because if you don't, you'll see that little crater under your toes.

7. When you have practiced enough to leave good footprints in the sand, try to Body Sense what it is that you're doing, so that you can implement all of the same motions into your regular running. I've also had people pretending they were running across hot coals in their bare feet. Whatever works . . .

8. When you are finally able to run the length of the sand without cratering, do this. At the end of most broad-jump pits there's a runaway that the broad jumpers use. Start at the end opposite the runway and run across the sand. When you get to the other side of the pit, continue running as if the runway were a continuing path of deep sand. Float across it the same way you floated across the sand pit and notice how lightly your feet touch the ground.

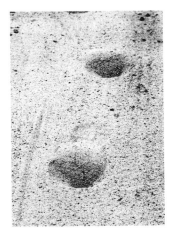

Figure 33—Making craters

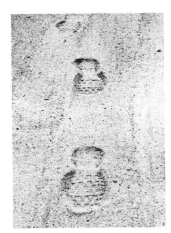

Figure 34—Leaving clean prints

What most people feel is an astounding reduction in the impact of their legs and feet with each stride. It will feel as though you're running on air. Lock in this memory so that you can retrieve it when you're out running.

SWING YOUR LEGS TO THE REAR

Another job of your lower body is to learn to "cooperate" with the force of the road coming at you—especially considering that that force *increases* as you run faster. This section will show you how to co-operate with that force so that it has little or no negative impact on your legs.

Every movement in T'ai Chi is balanced with a movement in the opposite direction. The same holds true for ChiRunning. The principle of Balance says that if a part of your body is moving forward, there needs to be another part of your body that is moving rearward to balance it. Since your upper body is moving forward (cooperating

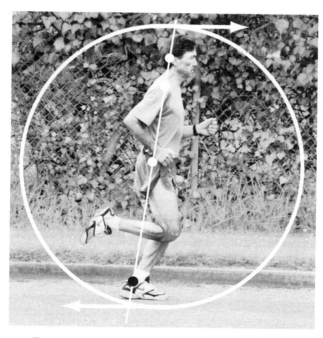

Figure 35—Upper body moves forward, lower body moves rearward

with the pull of gravity), your lower body is responsible for providing the necessary balance by moving in a rearward direction, and cooperating with the force of the road coming at you (see figure 35).

If you lift your knees and reach forward with each stride, your heels will strike in front of you and you'll be braking with every stride. That's what we call a forward swing of the legs, or reaching with your legs.

On the other hand, if you simply bend your knees (without lifting them) as your leg returns to your support position, your foot will come down on a midfoot strike under you instead of in front of you. This bending of the knees allows your stride to always remain behind your body, where it belongs. When your stride opens up behind you, your legs will be swinging *rearward* (the same direction as the road), and your stride will feel more fluid and balanced.

Exercise: Knee-Bending Exercise

Here's an exercise to help you bring all of the lower body focuses together. It's a drill used to help you learn to pick up your feet without picking up your knees. You'll be doing this exercise in three progressive steps: bending your knees, then leaning, then engaging your upper body.

Step 1: Bend your knees.

- Stand in a good posture stance, keeping your column in mind. Hold your arms at your sides with your elbows straight and your hands holding on to the sides of your legs.
- Run in place by keeping your knees down and gently picking up your heels behind you. Bend your knees enough to get your shins parallel to the ground (your leg will be bent at a right angle). Do not let yourself bend at the waist or lift your knees (that's why you're holding on to your legs with your hands). You should feel yourself landing on your midfoot, not on your toes. You should also not be pushing off with your toes (which causes you to bounce up and down). It's just a heel lift and a knee bend.

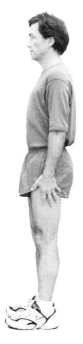

Figure 36—Bend knee exercise: hold onto your quads

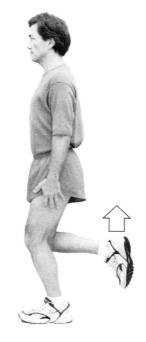

Figure 37—Run in place with knees down, heels up

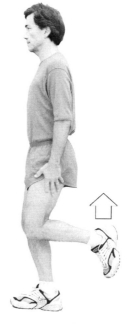

Figure 38—Land on your whole foot

- Keep your lower legs as limp as you can while doing this step. (This includes your toes, feet, ankles, and calves.)
- Run in place for a count of thirty knee bends.
- Stop and rest for thirty seconds.
- Repeat this step three times and try to get as relaxed as you can while doing it.

Step 2: Add a lean to the knee-bending exercise.

- Do Step 1 except this time you'll be tilting your Column while you're doing the exercise.

- Start running in place, drop your attention to the bottom of your feet. Keep your feet hitting at the bottom of your Column and then just let your Column tilt forward slightly. Don't change anything that you're doing with your body. Just add a slight tilt (only an inch or two), and remember to lean from your ankles. Let gravity pull your body forward for 20 feet. Be sure that you're not tensing your ankles at all as you lean. Remember to keep your lower legs limp.

Step 3: Add the arm swing.

- Repeat Step 2
- Find a spot on the ground about 10 yards from where you are starting, and when you pass that point, bend your elbows and swing your arms to the rear. If all goes well, you will feel yourself moving along, pulled forward by your lean. Remember to keep picking up your feet to keep up with your forward momentum. Visualize yourself moving along on a conveyor belt.

Practice your y'chi. If you want to practice your y'chi in this exercise, add this. Before you do the third step, while standing in place, focus your eyes on some spot or object in the distance. Train your vision on this point as if you were a guided missile, and don't break your gaze from the time you begin moving forward until you stop. Allow your visual connection with your "goal" to pull your body forward while you're moving through all the steps of the knee-bending exercise.

Remember, you're teaching your body to do something new, and you don't have to get it right the first time. Relax and try it again, as many times as it takes to feel the pull of gravity and the lift of your feet.

The reason why it's important to keep your knees down is because lifting your knees will bring your footstrike too far forward and into the territory where greater impact and heel striking occurs. If you keep your knees down, your foot will strike under or behind your center of gravity where it needs to, and your knees will swing forward but not come up.

THE MIDFOOT STRIKE:
DON'T RUN WITH THE BRAKES ON

Another benefit of leaning is that it changes where and how your feet strike the ground. Running with a vertical torso makes you have to reach forward with one leg while you push off with the other. This causes your foot to land in front of you with a heel strike as it hits the ground, which means you're essentially "putting on the brakes" with every stride. Your knee then becomes the transfer point between the force of your body moving forward and your foot, which is stopping. That's a lot of pressure being put on a joint that is not designed to withstand a huge amount of repetitive impact. Most people average 2,500 strides per mile, and each foot strike is estimated to be up to six times your body weight. If you're running at a 10:00-per-mile pace, it means that some multiple of your body weight is coming down on your knee 2,500 times every ten minutes! Knee injuries are by far the most common and the most debilitating of running injuries, and heel striking is a major culprit.

ChiRunning offers you an alternative to this physical abuse. By tilting your Column from your feet (not from your waist), you are essentially placing your center of mass *ahead* of your foot strike. Any physicist will tell you that when this occurs, you are no longer "braking" because your feet are landing in a midfoot strike and moving *toward the rear* when they strike the ground. This allows your legs to swing out behind you as soon as your feet touch the ground, radically reducing the amount of impact to your knees and quads. As soon as your feet hit the ground, they're gone . . . out the back. There's no braking, and you are truly cooperating with the force of the road coming at you.

The midfoot strike is exactly how it sounds. You're not landing on only the heel or the ball of the foot. Your whole foot lands, with the pressure equally balanced from front to back and side to side.

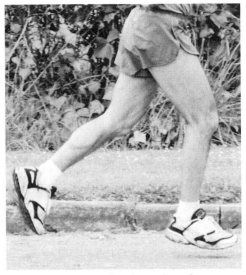

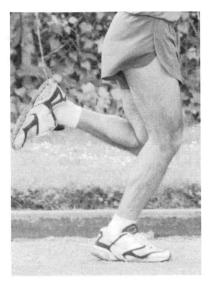

Figure 39—Leading leg relaxed   **Figure 40—Midfoot strike**

The slight forward lean and the midfoot strike creates the condition for your legs to fully relax and not be used for propulsion (figures 39 and 40). Your legs are only used for the momentary support between strides. After the support phase of your stride, your legs swing out behind you along with the force of the road. This is the ChiRunning approach to energy efficiency that sets it apart from other forms of running.

You'll get a great feel of the midfoot strike when you practice the sand pit and knee-bending exercises.

> **A Visualization: The Wheel:** Visualize yourself inside of a big wheel where the top of the wheel (your head) is moving forward and the bottom of the wheel (your foot) is moving to the rear as you roll down the road (see figure 35, page 91).
>
> You can also visualize your feet moving in circular patterns. Imagine your toes clipped into the pedals on a bike and you can only pull up on the pedals. In figure 41 you'll notice that the "wheels" of your feet are positioned slightly behind your body, unlike a bicycle, where the pedals are under your body.

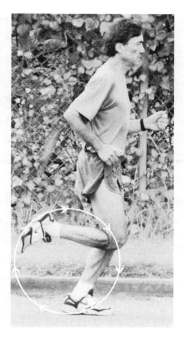

Figure 41—Circular feet

Pelvic Rotation

Okay, I know I often say that one thing or another is the most important thing about your running, but I mean it here. Learning to rotate your hips is the absolute, bottom-line key to good running form. Yes, everything else is important too, but your hips and pelvis are where energy-efficient running and injury prevention really happen. As you learn to rotate your pelvis you will seriously reduce the impact to everything below your waist, and your stride will take on a new level of smoothness you won't believe.

In the posture section, we had you engage your core muscles to level your pelvis. We mentioned three reasons why this is so important and explained the first: to maintain a straight Column while running (or walking). In this section we'll continue discussing our reasons for leveling the pelvis with points 2 and 3: to keep the pelvis level while it rotates, and to create a more powerful connection between the pelvis and legs, unifying the movement of the whole lower body.

In the ChiRunning technique your legs swing to the rear. This movement of your legs creates a rotation in your lower body. Your upper body remains stable (with no rotation) and your lower body, including your pelvis, rotates around its central axis. When your core is engaged, your legs become an *extension* of your pelvis, keeping the origin of movement in your center, not the other way around. Your legs then passively follow the rotation of your pelvis while also providing support during each foot strike. In T'ai Chi, all of the movement of your legs originates from your center (your pelvic area).

If your core is not engaged, the connection between your pelvis and your legs is lost and the power from your core is cut off. This, in turn, makes your legs have to do all the work, which is what we're trying to get away from.

There are two main ways runners underuse their pelvis: not rotating the pelvis while running, and not leveling the pelvis (engaging the core muscles) while running. You need to Body Sense for yourself which you are, but in general men tend to hold too much tension in their pelvic area, creating stiffness, and women tend to have too little core strength in their pelvis, which leaves that area unstable.

If your pelvis does not rotate, it means your legs have to swing entirely from your hip joints, which puts a lot of strain on them. Running faster can increase the pull on the ligaments and tendons in your hips and cause long-term problems. Also, if your pelvis is immobile, it's generally because you are holding tension in your glutes, your quads, or your lower back muscles. All of that tightness in your spine and pelvis inhibits the flow of chi up and down your spine and prevents your legs from swinging freely when you run. A much more efficient way of stabilizing your pelvis when you run is to engage your core muscles by leveling your pelvis. You can then relax all those poor, overused glutes and lower back muscles.

Also, if your pelvis does not rotate (because you hold tension there), you'll absorb the force of the road with your knees, quads, hips, or lower back. Allowing your pelvis to rotate allows the road to move right on by, without sending any of that force into your body.

If your hips and pelvis are too loose, more often than not your pelvis will move laterally (side to side) when you run, rather than rotating around the axis of your spine. If you've seen me in classes, you might remember my Mae West impersonation. Think of how a fashion model walks down the runway with swaying hips: that's an exaggeration of what I see in those with too little core stability. In this case, the pelvis is at the mercy of what the legs do, which makes your lower back and hips vulnerable to injury because of too much unsupported movement.

THE PIVOT POINT: T12/L1

In order for your pelvis to rotate, your spine has to twist. The point along your spine where the twist happens is at T12/L1. We call it the Pivot Point. This is the place on your spine where the curve of your upper (thoracic) spine meets the curve of your lower (lumbar) spine.

You can find T12/L1 by putting your fingers on your lowest rib and following that rib with your fingers back to the spine. In ChiRunning, we say that the lower body begins at the Pivot Point because it is the point from which all of the motion of your lower body begins. What this means (and it may sound a bit strange) is that your legs don't just swing from your hips, they swing from T12/L1, which gives you a much better range of motion. Allowing everything below your Pivot Point to swing allows your shoulders and upper body to always face forward.

Figure 44 shows the leg swinging to the rear pulling

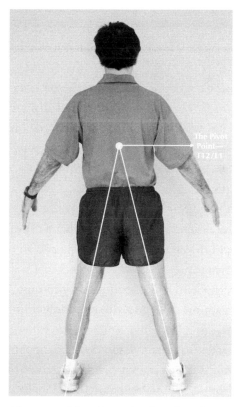

Figure 42—Your lower body swings from your Pivot Point

the hip with it. Relaxing your lower back allows your spine to twist more easily; this increases the rotation of your pelvis, which then allows your stride to increase behind you. Put your attention on your Pivot Point and notice that everything below that point is moving and everything above that point is not. Whenever you walk or run, become aware of the twist of your spine.

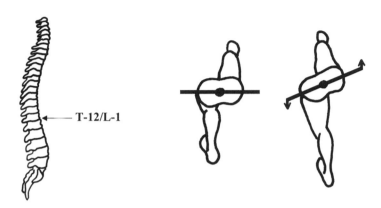

Figure 43—The spinal column   Figure 44—Pelvis not rotating and
                                    pelvis rotating

Each time your foot hits the ground, your hip is pulled rearward by your leg, which then rotates your pelvis, and your entire lower body swings from your Pivot Point. Don't force your hip to swing to the rear, just let it happen. Train your hips and lower back to relax so that your stride can lengthen behind you as you run faster.

Here's a fun exercise that will help you get a clear sense of what pelvic rotation feels like. It works much better if you do it with a friend.

Exercise: The Pool Running Drill

Remember when you were a kid and you were at the local pool? Remember when you wanted to be first in line for the diving board or slide? What did you do . . . that's right, you ran for that first spot but it was *always* foiled by the lifeguard yelling, "Hey you . . . WALK!!!" At which point you went into the fastest walk you could possible sustain without losing any ground speed.

Have your friend pretend to be the lifeguard. Go out in the street and pretend you're that kid out of your past running across the pool deck. Start running, and after about 10 yards, have your friend yell, "Hey you . . . WALK!!!" at which point you'll try to do the same thing that the kid in your past did. That's right, drop into a very fast walk as if your life depended on you getting to the diving board first.

The first thing you'll notice is that when you walk fast, your upper body leans into the direction you're heading, while your hips swing like crazy. When you're walking this way, there should be no mistake about whether or not your pelvis is rotating. You should also get a clear sense of your shoulders always facing forward as you lead with your upper body.

Keep walking fast for a short distance and feel your pelvis rotating as you move forward. When you have a distinct feeling of your pelvis and hips swinging allow yourself to break into an easy jog *while continuing to feel your pelvis rotate.* If you're doing it right, your running should take on a nice sense of relaxation and flow.

You'll find another pelvic rotation exercise in Chapter 8 in the Body Looseners section (see page 196).

In ChiRunning, it ain't the muscle, it's the motion—and the motion comes from gravity, the force of the road, and allowing your pelvis to do its job of swinging.

Visualization: Upper and Lower Body Movement: Stable Above, Swinging Below: Imagine your whole lower body is suspended like a chandelier at the Pivot Point. Your upper body is aimed in the direction you are heading, cooperating with gravity, aligned in the direction of your forward motion, and your lower body is doing all the swinging.

We've discovered in teaching ChiWalking that it is easier to learn pelvic rotation while walking than while running. Once you can feel this sensation in your walking you'll be able to integrate it into your running. While running you want to allow your hips to rotate as fully as they do during this exercise. For some advanced work get a Chubby Checker record and do the twist!!

Upper Body Form Focuses

It don't mean a thing if it ain't got that swing.
—Duke Ellington

In the ChiRunning technique your upper body has a lot to contribute
to your running. Think of your body as a team of two, working together to help you run. This "team" consists of your upper body and
your lower body. The more you can get both partners to cooperate
and work together, the easier the workload will feel. When the upper
body is doing its fair share, you can reduce your overall effort significantly.

The upper body focuses consist of arm swing and upper body position.

ARM SWING

Let's talk about the physics of your arm swing. Basically, your arms
(and legs too, for that matter) are pendulums. Your arms swing from
your shoulders and your legs swing from your hips. The law of the
pendulum states that any pendulum of a given length will always
swing at the same rate (swings per minute). If you want a pendulum
to swing faster, you can either force it faster, or you can shorten it. If
you want your arms and legs to swing faster there are two ways to get
that to happen. The first way is to force them to swing faster with
your muscles, which would obviously increase your muscle usage and
fuel consumption. The second way is to shorten your pendulum by
simply bending your elbow (or knee.) This makes your arm pendulum about half as long as it was when it was straight, allowing it to
swing faster.

Try this demonstration of the pendulum effect with your arms.

- Stand upright and let your arms hang at your sides.
- Keeping your elbows locked in this straight position, swing
  them as fast as you can.

- After about five seconds, bend your elbows to a 90° angle, but keep them swinging fast for a few seconds and then stop.

Did you feel a noticeable difference in effort when you bent your elbows? Well, the same holds true for your legs. They'll swing more easily if they're bent.

Here's a list of things to help to improve your arm swing.

- **Bend your elbows** at a 90° angle and allow your arms to swing from your shoulders in a relaxed way. A bent arm will always swing more easily than a straight arm. Don't pump your arms (opening and closing your 90° angle). The best way to tell if you're holding your arms in the right position is to never let your hands fall below your waistband. If you're not used to holding your hands higher, it might feel hard at first. But once your arms get used to being comfortably held in this position, you won't notice any extra work going on and your arms will swing much more freely. Focus on the tips of your elbows when practicing your arm swing, not on your entire arm. It's psychologically *much* easier to swing a small body part (your elbow) than it is to swing a large body part (your arm).

- **Swing your arms to the *rear***, not forward. Imagine that you're trying to elbow someone behind you, instead of trying to punch someone in front of you. Swinging your elbows to the rear creates a counter-balance to the forward lean of your body. The range of motion of your arm swing should be as follows: your fingers should come back to your ribs (figure 45) and your elbows should come forward only to your ribs (figure 46). If your elbows swing in front of your ribs, it will cause your legs to swing too far forward, creating more heelstrike. If you'd really like to swing your arms forward, save it until you're either sprinting or running uphill (see Chapter 7).

- **Don't cross your centerline with your hands.** Your forearms should swing slightly across your body, but your hands should not cross your centerline. If they do, it creates too much side-to-side motion in your upper body. Just imagine you're holding a volley-

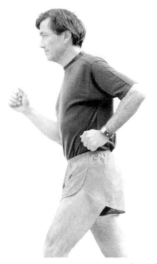 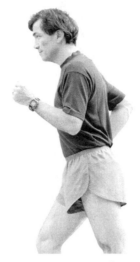

Figure 45—Arm swing: hands   Figure 46—Arm swing: elbows
to your ribs   to your ribs

ball between your palms and don't let your hands get any closer
than the width of the ball.

- **Relax your hands.** Hold them with your fingers curled inward
  and your thumbs on top. I heard someone once describe it as
  pretending that you just caught a butterfly and you don't want to
  crush it. (White knuckles are a definite no-no.) Your wrists should
  be straight and not bent backward. Basically, chi will not flow
  through tight joints. And, if your joints are tight, it means that
  your muscles are working more than is necessary.

HEAD, NECK, AND SHOULDERS

Here are a few things worth mentioning regarding what to do with
this area of the body while running.

- **Keep your shoulders low and relaxed** as you swing your arms.
  Don't use your shoulders to swing your arms. Use your hat, not
  your shoulders, to keep your ears warm. It is important that your
  shoulders hold as little tension as possible. I've met *way* too many

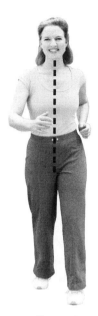

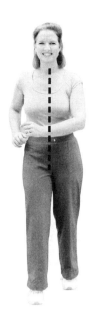

Figure 47—Correct arm swing: hands should never cross your centerline

Figure 48—Incorrect arm swing: hands crossing the centerline

runners with tightness in their neck and shoulders from holding their elbows out away from their sides. Let your elbows pass close to your ribs. This helps your neck and shoulders to relax. If you have a tendency to hold tension in your shoulders, drop your hands to your sides every now and then and let them just dangle at your sides for a few strides.

- **Shoulders always face forward.** Don't swing your shoulders. Pretend that your shoulders are like the two headlights of a car and they're always pointing forward. This will allow your lower body its full range of rotation. If your upper body rotates when you run, you'll end up shortening your stride length and lose a lot of efficiency.

- **Lengthen the back of your neck** (as described in the Posture section). This will hold your posture nice and tall with each stride. If your chin juts forward, it throws your whole posture off. (See "Posture," page 61).

- **Be sure to look around** when you run. Relax your neck and take in your surroundings every now and then . . . there's more to life than trying to remember a gazillion focuses.

Brief Review

Before you start to run, on the following pages are two sequences of photos showing incorrect and correct form. The best place to get this visual and really see ChiRunning in action is on the DVD.

Let's start with what happens when you're not running correctly. In figure 49 you'll notice my head is directly over my feet, I'm bent at the waist and my chin is up. In figure 50 I am reaching forward with my leg and dorsiflexing my ankle, which causes a heel strike. I'm also reaching forward with my arms. In figure 51 you'll get a great view of a heel strike (putting on the brakes). In figure 52 I'm lifting my knee. In figure 54 you'll see how I am bent forward at the waist and my hips are behind my foot strike. This is *not* the way it should be, and each thing I have pointed out has potential for injury.

Now, we'll review the ChiRunning form. In figure 55 you'll see that my Column is lined up. I've lengthened the back of my neck and my chin is down. In figure 59 you'll notice my knees are low, I don't dorsiflex, and my toe is lower than my heel (no chance of a heel strike). My elbow is swinging to the rear and my chin is down. In figures 58 and 60 you'll see a clear midfoot strike supporting a one-legged posture stance.

Over time, you'll become your own expert at being able to see what is correct and what is not correct.

GEARS, CADENCE, AND STRIDE LENGTH

Utilizing gears in your stride is a great tool that will allow beginners to run without getting as tired and seasoned runners to improve energy efficiency and speed at the same time. Gears are as important to your running as they are to bikes and cars. In running you change gears by changing your stride length. The faster you go, the higher the gear, and in the case of running it means leaning more and increasing the length of your stride. When you run slowly (in a low gear), you should have a very short stride.

Incorrect running form:

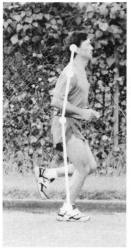

Figure 49

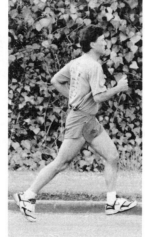

Figure 50

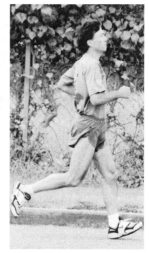

Figure 51

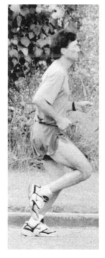

Figure 52

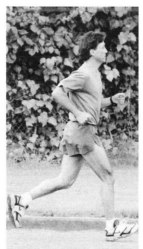

Figure 53

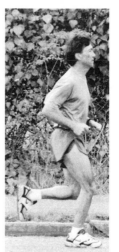

Figure 54

Now, let's see what it looks like when you do it right:

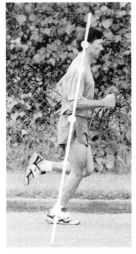

Figure 55

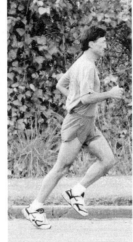

Figure 56

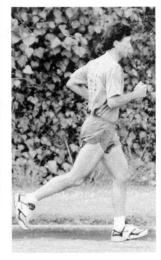

Figure 57

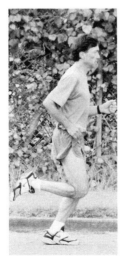

Figure 58

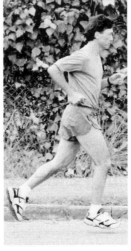

Figure 59

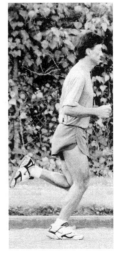

Figure 60

Gears are also used to reduce your perceived effort level while running uphill. If you drive your car up a hill in high gear, you'll burn much more gas than if you shift to a lower gear. We'll discuss this in the section in Chapter 7, "Hills, Trails, and Treadmills."

What *doesn't* change is your cadence, the rate at which your feet touch the ground. Do the math. If you maintain a steady cadence but increase your lean, your stride will lengthen naturally and you'll pick up speed. Speed is not a factor of working harder. This is the opposite of power running, where runners generally open up their stride by lifting their knees and reaching forward with their legs. If you do this, you are swinging your legs *into* the force of the road coming at you, which increases your impact with the ground.

Let's use the example of riding a ten-speed bike to illustrate how cadence applies to your running. Most competitive cyclists try to maintain a pedaling cadence of about 85–90 rpm. This allows them to maintain a steady perceived effort level no matter which gear they are using. If they want to go faster, they simply keep the same cadence, shift to a higher gear . . . and speed happens. This way of combining cadence with gears also works with running.

An important point that I would like to emphasize here is how cadence and stride length (or gears) work together to affect your perceived rate of exertion. When these two team up, magic happens. Once you are able to run at a steady cadence in all gears, your perceived rate of exertion will be greatly reduced because you are only increasing your abdominal muscle usage (to maintain the lean), not your leg muscle usage. As you improve your ChiRunning skills you won't have to think about adjusting your stride length; it will happen naturally, as a function of leaning and relaxing your legs. In essence, your legs aren't working harder as you run faster. In fact, the more you can allow your entire lower body to swing from the Pivot Point, the faster you will go.

GEARS

For simplicity's sake, in ChiRunning we speak about every runner having four different gears. With each successive gear comes an increase in the length of your stride. If you've done any running at all, you should be able to relate to the four gears I'm about to describe.

- **First gear** is your lowest gear and your slowest speed. It's the speed to use for your warm-up.
- **Second gear** is the speed you would run if you were going out for an average training run. It's an easy, conversational pace you run when you're doing longer distances.
- **Third gear** is a distance-race pace, meaning any distance over a mile. Whatever distance you would race, this would be the speed you would try to average. It's at the high end of your aerobic capacity, so you'll be a little more out of breath.
- **Fourth gear** is sprint or anaerobic pace. You could not carry on a conversation at this pace. In an anaerobic state, your lungs cannot provide enough oxygen for your muscles to sustain this speed indefinitely. It's only for short distances.

Each of these four gears is distinctly different from the others, and when you're running, you should be able to feel which gear you're in at any given time.

Gears in a Nutshell
- Slower speed = less lean = shorter stride = lower gear
- Higher speed = more lean = longer stride = higher gear
- As you lean your body forward, your stride opens up out the back
- Cadence always remains the same

EXERCISE: INCREMENTAL LEANING FOR GEARS
Ask a friend to help you practice this lean. Stand in your best posture and have your friend put their fingertip 1 inch in front of your nose. Then, lean from your ankles (keeping your Column straight), until your nose just touches your friend's finger. This will give you the Body Sense of what 1 inch of lean feels like.

Each of your four gears is approximately one additional inch of lean from vertical. You'll see from the leaning exercise you've just done that 1 inch of lean is *very small*. This should show you that it is easy to lean too much. If you're leaning too much, you'll be off balance and your lower leg muscles will engage to hold you in your lean. Always work to balance yourself in your lean so that your lower legs can remain relaxed.

With each additional inch of lean it is important to remember to do two things: level your pelvis (which keeps your Column aligned) while allowing it to rotate *more*. Remember to keep lengthening the back of your neck to prevent your chin from coming up as you increase your lean.

When you slow down and drop to a lower gear, remember to *shorten your stride* so you can maintain a steady cadence.

CADENCE

I never paid much attention to my cadence before I started developing the ChiRunning technique. It was what it was. As I ran faster my legs turned over faster, which I expected. But, once I began to study the physics of efficiency, I realized that I was doing it all backward. Instead of having my cadence go *faster* as I picked up speed, it felt easier to let my cadence *stay the same* and lengthen my stride as I picked up speed. By doing this, my body adjusted to running at the same cadence no matter what the speed.

Your cadence is measured as the number of strides per minute that *one leg* takes. So a cadence of 85 would mean that your right leg takes 85 strides every minute.

We have found on average, that people's cadence, before learning ChiRunning is between 80 and 83. If your cadence is slower than 85 strides per minute, your feet stay in contact with the ground longer, which means that your legs are supporting your body weight for a longer period of time. Conversely, if your cadence is above 85 strides per minute, you'll spend significantly less time on your feet, saving valuable energy. However, if your cadence is above 90 spm, it could be because your pelvis is not rotating, causing your turnover to increase as you run faster. This faster turnover works fine for sprinters and elite middle distance runners, but it is a very inefficient way for anyone else to run because of the increased workload to the quads and hamstrings to turn the legs over faster.

STRIDE LENGTH

A comment we often hear from students about stride length and cadence is that in ChiRunning their stride feels shorter and quicker than they're used to, especially at slower speeds. I agree, because one of the most common and significant problems I see in runners is that many, if not most, have too long a stride length and too slow a cadence when they're running slowly. This is very inefficient and tiring to the body.

When you're running in first gear, your feet should be moving in a small circular motion, like you're pedaling a little kid's bicycle. As you increase your speed, this wheel will increase in size. You'll find an extraordinary example of this on the ChiRunning DVD in the Cadence Lesson. The screen is split into four quadrants with the runner holding a steady cadence while running in each of the four gears. In it you'll see, that as my lean increases, so does my stride length (and the size of my "wheel"). You'll also see that the *cadence never changes*, no matter what speed I'm running.

As we have already mentioned in the "Pelvic Rotation" section, the increase in your stride length will come from increasing your pelvic rotation, which in turn allows your legs to swing out behind you.

THE METRONOME: A GREAT TRAINING TOOL

The first step in learning to run in different gears is to practice maintaining a steady cadence. I'm not big on having lots of training gizmos, but I would have to say that I have learned more from running with a metronome than I have from any other device, book, or coach. Find a metronome on the ChiRunning website.

The metronome will teach you how to run at a steady cadence, and the result is that your stride length will naturally decrease and increase depending on your speed.

Here's how to work with a metronome:

- Without the metronome, go out on a run, and once you are warmed up and settled into your stride, count the number of steps your right leg takes over a one-minute period.
- After you figure out what your current cadence is, set your metronome to beep at your current cadence. Then run with your metronome for a week just to get used to matching your footfall with the beat.
- After one week, if your beginning cadence is lower than 85, increase your setting by one beep per minute and run with the new beat for a week. Repeat this increase weekly until you're up to 85–90 spm. Let's say your current cadence is 78 spm. If you start off running with your metronome set at 78 spm and increase it by one beat each week, it will take you seven weeks to get up to 85 spm . . . now *that's* Gradual Progress.

The real beauty of the metronome is that if you match your footfall to the beep then your stride length will naturally decrease or increase in length depending on the speed you are running.

Which cadence is best for you? If you're tall or long-legged, your cadence should be closer to 85 spm. If you're shorter and have little stubby legs like mine, you should shoot for a cadence closer to 90 spm. Those little legs need to turn over faster.

Would anyone like to waltz? Once you can run at a steady cadence and match the metronome with your stride, we recommend that you run with your metronome beeping once every three strides. Here's why. If you set your metronome to beep 90 bpm and you're matching your right leg to the beat, you might inadvertently overemphasize the motion of your right leg. Since the ChiRunning technique is all about learning balance, we suggest that you run with a waltz tempo and have the metronome beep every third stride. This way, the "downbeat" will match your right foot and then, three strides later, it'll match your *left* foot, and so on. It's just like waltzing: *right*, two, three, *left*, two, three, *right*, two, three . . .

To accomplish this, take your current cadence, multiply it by .66, and then set your metronome at the resulting number. For example, if your cadence is 90 spm, you'd set your metronome to 60 bpm and run to a three-count. When I'm running, I really prefer the gliding smoothness of a waltz to a two-step.

Remember, once you have gotten your cadence to where it should be, your cadence *never* changes, no matter how fast or slow you are running. Practice keeping an even tempo of 85–90 steps per minute. I set mine at 90 and start off running at a slow pace and very short stride-length, which gradually lengthens as I lean more. My challenge is to maintain a cadence of 90 whether I'm leaning a little or a lot. I've been using my metronome for years and it has helped me immensely in learning how to vary my stride length at different speeds.

Let's Go Running

That's it—those are all the Form Focuses. And here is where you finally get to start running. We know that it might seem a bit overwhelming, but don't worry. We're going to get you started running, and in Chapter 5 we will take you through specific lessons and help you learn the ChiRunning technique over time, whether you're just starting a running program or incorporating ChiRunning into an established running routine.

This next exercise for starting to run is what you do the first time you try ChiRunning, whether you're a beginner or a veteran. Since it's your first time out, we've kept this first section simple. You'll find this section on the ChiRunning DVD as well. Review it before you go out for your first run.

This is the sequence of focuses I use in my classes, which has proven itself with the test of time. Let your mind direct your body and let your body feel the focuses. You'll remember each Form Focus better if you can Body Sense each one as you do it.

REVIEW THE FOCUSES BEFORE YOUR RUN
1. Begin by practicing your posture stance.
   • Stand with your feet parallel and hip width apart, feeling your feet balanced front to back, side to side, and right to left.

- Straighten your upper body by lengthening the back of your neck.
- Level your pelvis.
- Adjust your hips—connect the dots (shoulders, hips, ankles).
- Feel your Column from your head to your feet.
- Drop your chin and check to see if you can see your shoelaces.

2. Next, find something to lean against and do your leaning exercise to remind yourself what it feels like to fall forward.
   - Stand one shoe length away from a fence, wall or tree, facing it.
   - Engage your "C" shape (your Column).
   - Fall forward a few times, pushing yourself back upright each time.
   - Keep your ankles relaxed and the pressure on the bottoms of your feet evenly distributed the entire time.

3. Walk around for a few minutes to practice picking up your feet.
   - Shake out your legs and keep your lower legs limp
   - Maintain your best posture.
   - Pick each foot up higher than the opposite ankle with each step.
   - There should not be any pressure under the ball of your foot as you walk. (Pretend you're sneaking up on someone.)

HOW TO START YOUR RUN

1. Stand with your best posture and set up your Column.
2. Practice a few one-legged posture stances on each leg before taking off.
3. Bend your arms to 90° and relax your shoulders.
4. Begin running slowly with a very short stride length. Your elbows should be swinging gently to the rear. (Run so slow that your breath rate hardly increases.)
5. Once you begin running, pretend that you're not running. That's right—imagine that you're just practicing a bunch of one-legged posture stances, one after another. Every time your foot touches the ground, you're landing in a one-legged posture stance. You should feel yourself landing on your midfoot, not your heel. Run this way for a few minutes and don't think about any other Focuses, or that you're even running. It's just you doing your one-legged

posture stances, and every time your foot lands on the ground, you are connecting the dots (shoulders, hips, ankles) and feeling your Column.

6. Run this way, with a short stride, until you feel that you can maintain a nice, straight posture line (Column) while running slowly.

7. Now it's time to use the three steps of engaging your lean.
   - Step 1: Check in with your posture line.
   - Step 2: Drop your attention to the bottoms of your feet.
   - Step 3: Keep your feet hitting at the base of your Column and let your whole posture line fall forward, slightly in front (about one inch off of vertical) of where your feet are hitting.

   Increase your lean by only a small amount and balance yourself in this new angle of lean. Let your legs swing to the rear.

8. Hold this new angle of lean for fifteen to thirty seconds and then let yourself come back upright to your original position. You should feel your speed decrease when you do this. At this point, most people express surprise upon feeling themselves slow down, because they were unaware that they had picked up their speed when they increased their lean. If you feel this slowdown, it's your body telling you that you had accelerated *without using your legs to do so*. It's all in the lean.

9. Do frequent check-ins to see if your Column is straight and that your foot is still hitting at the bottom. Repeat the exercise of increasing your lean and holding it for fifteen to thirty seconds, alternating with returning back to an upright position for the same amount of time. Do this leaning exercise ten times and then take a walking break. When you're leaning, your upper body should be slightly ahead of your foot strike. If it were a race between your head and your feet, your head would *always* cross the finish line first.

10. While you're walking, focus on maintaining your Column and relaxing your body.

In the next chapter we'll show you how to use Gradual Progress to learn the ChiRunning technique and incorporate all the ChiRunning focuses into your running program.

FOCUS LIST

Here is a complete list of focuses to refer back to before heading out on a run. Pick one or two for every workout.

POSTURE

Align your feet and legs

Soften your knees

Balance your feet (left/right, front/back, inside/outside)

Lengthen the back of your neck and drop your chin

Level your pelvis

Relax your glutes

Create your Column (shoulders, hips, ankles aligned)

Feel your feet at the bottom of your Column

Look for your shoelaces

One-legged posture stance

The "C" shape

Feel your Column with each foot strike

Relax everything but your lower abs

LEAN

Three steps to engage lean

1. Check in with your posture
2. Drop your focus to your feet
3. Keep your feet landing where they are and let your Column fall in front of where your feet are hitting

Relax lower legs and ankles

Lengthen the back of your neck and lead with your forehead

Land midfoot

Upper body ahead of your feet

Balance in the "window of lean"

Feel your lower abs engage more as you lean more

Your lean is your gas pedal

LOWER BODY

Legs

    Start off with short stride

    Swing legs to the rear

    Let your hip swing back with your leg

    Rotate legs medially (toward your midline) to point feet forward

Lower Legs

    Bend your knees

    Limp lower legs: calves, shins, ankles, feet, toes

    Heels up, knees down

    Soften knees

    Passive lower legs

Feet and Ankles

    Feet point forward

    Circular feet with wheels at the ends of your legs

    Lift your ankles

    Heels up, toes down

    Peel foot off the ground

    Midfoot strike

Pelvic Rotation

    Feel your Pivot Point at T12/L1

    Level your pelvis

    Allow pelvic rotation to happen—relax and don't force anything

    Entire lower body rotates below Pivot Point

UPPER BODY

Arm Swing

    Bend your elbows to 90° (don't pump)

    Curl fingers, with thumbs on top; relax hands

    Hands always held above your waistline

    Hands don't cross your centerline

Swing elbows to the rear

Shoulders fall forward, elbows counter-balance rearward

Head, Neck, Shoulders

Keep shoulders low and relaxed

Shoulders always face forward

Lengthen back of neck; lengthen spine

Lead with your forehead

Y'chi directs energy forward through the eyes

Breathing

Belly-breathe—inhale through nose, exhale through mouth by pulling your belly in

Match breath rate to cadence: exhale for two steps, inhale for one

Nose-breathe if possible

CADENCE, GEARS, AND STRIDE LENGTH

Cadence

Work toward a range between 85 and 90 spm with a metronome

If your current cadence is below 85 spm, start there and increase your cadence by one stride per minute each week until you reach 85

Gears and Stride Length

First gear

- 1-inch lean
- Shortest stride length
- Warm-up pace
- Breath rate barely increases

Second gear

- 2-inch lean
- Medium stride length
- Conversational/training pace
- Aerobic pace

Third gear

- 3-inch lean

- Race pace
- Longest stride length
- High end of aerobic pace

Fourth gear

- 4-inch lean
- Sprint pace
- Third-gear stride length
- Anaerobic pace
- Arms swing forward (not to the rear)
- Drive with your hips (not your legs)
- Slight increase in cadence but not in stride length
- Engage the "C" shape more *and* relax hips and legs more

CHAPTER FIVE

How to Learn ChiRunning

If you are reaching deeper within yourself with compassion, patience, perseverance, and forgiveness as you work toward the goal or victory, then you will learn and grow.
—MICHAEL TAMURA, *YOU ARE THE ANSWER*

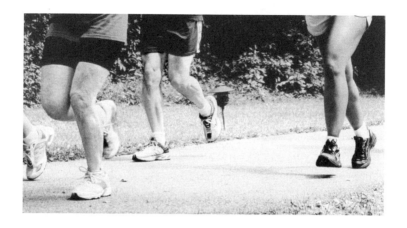

What you will find in this section are ten lessons to learn ChiRunning, a few helpful tips for learning, and the stages you can expect to go through in this process. Whether you're a beginning runner or a seasoned vet, we suggest you take yourself through these ten lessons, in the order presented. After many years of teaching, I have found that this sequence is the best way to incorporate the focuses into your running. After the ten lessons I have listed a group of paired Focuses that are great to practice together. Use this list once you feel comfortable with the ten lessons.

On our website at www.chirunning.com you can find an online training log and training programs for beginners to advanced runners, training for a 5K, 10K, half marathon, or marathon. In each of these training programs we'll teach you how to run the distance while developing your ChiRunning skills at the same time.

In Chapter 6, "Program Development," we'll talk more about various kinds of runs and creating a running program for yourself, but in this chapter we simply focus on the lessons to learn ChiRunning.

Here are some important tips about learning:

- **Non-identification—getting your ego out of the way.** Non-identification is a phrase that basically means putting aside all your personal ideas and preferences and responding to what "is" in any situation. For example, you're out running with your marathon training group and you feel particularly slow that day. Your ego will first disapprove of what "is" (that you are slower than your group) and will want you to keep up with your group so that it doesn't feel bad about itself. You, on the other hand, really need to listen to your body, run at whatever pace is right for you, be with your technique and find the speed when and if it happens.

  Every time you go out for a run you need to respond to your environmental conditions: hills, rough terrain, cold, wind, and so on, plus your bodily conditions: fatigue, muscle tension or soreness, adrenaline, various emotional states, lack of sleep—whatever is going on in your mind and body. In most cases there is a best way to handle the external conditions and/or your particular state of being. If you can just observe the situation from a neutral place and without judgment, your assessment of the situation will be more accurate, as will your response. ChiRunning is all about objectively observing the conditions and responding in the way that is most appropriate.

  When I'm out trail running, for instance, I can run much better and more efficiently if I go with the flow of the trail instead of fighting it. When I'm running up a steep hill, I don't get bummed out that there's a lot of work ahead. I relax my legs, which shortens my stride, making the hill easier to negotiate. I don't resist the hill; I make friends with it and let it show me what to do.

  Non-identification also means making *friends* with injuries by letting them tell you what you're doing wrong. When people tell me that they've had a bad run, it's music to my ears. If I ask the right questions about why they considered the run bad, I can pinpoint the weak spot in their technique and guide them to the necessary correction. If you look at your challenging or difficult runs in this way, you won't be as compelled to call them "bad runs." Instead, you could tell your friends that you had a good "running lesson" today.

- **Start simple.** Remember the principle of Gradual Progress: the best things take patience and perseverance. Give yourself lots of time and space to learn this stuff; don't try to take on too much at first. Go slowly and celebrate your small successes. Do only as much as you can do well, and don't worry about the rest—it'll come. When you feel comfortable with one Focus, add another. Always try to get a clear Body Sense of what you are focusing on before you try to add more. You'll be practicing the principle of Gradual Progress by taking small steps and letting your knowledge grow in a steady and solid way.

- **Have a clear image of what you're supposed to do.** Read and reread the specific Focus you're working on until you have a clear understanding of the concept and what you will be doing when you go out to run. View the lesson on the DVD. If it's a Focus that you can practice indoors, by all means do it a few times before you head out the door. The more thorough you are in the beginning stages, the better your chances are of developing a beautiful, smooth running form.

- **Consistency.** They say it's hard to teach an old dog new tricks. That's why your body, just like the old dog, learns best with repetition. Learning new habits of movement takes consistency and persistence, and the more often you practice the Form Focuses, the more quickly your body will learn them. I suggest a minimum running program of three days a week to start. When you're building a body memory, it's best not to wait too long between practice sessions because it saves you from having to start from scratch each time you go out.

- **Get a second opinion.** It is sometimes hard to tell if you're moving correctly. One way to solve this problem is to learn ChiRunning with a running partner. If both of you are learning the Focuses together, you can act as each other's "eyes" and offer observations or suggestions on what you see.

Another suggestion is to have your running videotaped so you can see if you're really doing what you think you're doing. The ideal place to do this is at your local high school track. Run the curved section at one end of the track while a friend films you from the infield (under the goalpost is best). This is a great training aid, because it allows you to see a side view of your running form. Borrow a video camera if you have to—it's worth it.

A third option is to look at your reflection when you run past a large glass storefront window. Just don't get caught fixing your hair.

Learning to use the ChiRunning focuses is much like learning to play a musical instrument. First you learn to play individual notes. Then, when you have that down, you learn to play lines and phrases of music, eventually playing an entire piece. As you perfect your playing technique you eventually get to a place where you can play without reading the music. And when you master your instrument, you and the instrument become an open channel for the music to pour through, and you can express your feelings through the music.

THE STAGES OF LEARNING EFFORTLESS, INJURY-FREE RUNNING

In ChiRunning we put before you the possibility, the golden ring of an idea, that you can run effortlessly and injury-free. Is this possible?

We believe the answer is yes. It is possible to run injury-free, barring accidents that can happen in everyday life and everyday running. And yes, when you get to a certain level with ChiRunning and into "the zone" of where you feel it all come together, ChiRunning can feel amazingly effortless; as many people have said, "It's like I could run forever."

Running injury-free and effortlessly are "ruling ideas" that you can, and should, focus on in every run. I do. In every run I'm asking myself, "How can I do this with less effort, with less strain?" That question will lead you on the path to injury-free and effortless running.

We know, however, there are often stages you must go through before ChiRunning really gives you that effortless feeling (although we do get many reports of people who get the effortless feeling very quickly and who report immediate pain relief from current injuries).

STAGE ONE: BEGINNER'S MIND

This stage is when you first open up to the possibility that you can learn a new way to run and that this new way is actually a good way for you to run. This is the stage of suspended disbelief, or in Buddhist terms, beginner's mind.

In Stage One, it is important to understand the underlying principles of ChiRunning, such as; when your spine is aligned, you will move more easily. Another principle that needs to be understood for effortless and injury-free running to "happen" is that efficient movement comes from your core muscles, not the muscles in your legs. We are so used to being told that strong legs are the answer to efficient running that when we're told to totally relax our legs, it is a huge mind and body shift away from how we normally move.

A short stride is also hard to accept. It just seems that we should reach as far as we can with our legs to gobble up more ground. But in doing so we are working harder than necessary and making ourselves injury-prone. This is the story of my wife, Katherine: "I never had an easy time with Danny teaching me to run—you know, the husband-wife thing. And his short, quick steps actually annoyed me. It looked like it was *more* effort to be so sprightly. But finally, over the years, I tried the short stride on my own, aided by the metronome, which forced me to quicken and shorten my stride, and I realized why I had suffered back pain for so many years." Leaning is another aspect of ChiRunning that may require "suspended disbelief," as is the fact that you may not be leaning when it feels like you are. So if you're willing to experiment, you can get through Stage One and move on to Stage Two.

STAGE TWO: EFFORTING

There are two types of effort you may have to make: an effort to focus your mind and an effort to move your body into the correct positioning.

Let's take your posture as an example. Since most people do have some posture issues, this is a place where you will need to remember (which is a mind focus) to practice being aligned, while physically engaging muscles that may not have been used in a while to create alignment. When the muscles that hold your posture in proper alignment become strong and when your body can maintain that alignment without your mind telling it to, good posture will become effortless. You may need to make a variety of changes that require mental and physical effort.

STAGE THREE: RELAX

Relaxation is a major component to effortless and injury-free running. Learning to relax can be an effort! It can be hard to relax your ankles, your glutes, your shoulders, and your legs. All this relaxing can take a lot of mental effort, but again, our bodies can learn quickly, especially when something feels good. Pretty soon relaxing becomes effortless and makes your running more effortless as well. But it is Stage Four that will finally get you to injury-free and effortless running.

STAGE FOUR: PLAY

Once you're ChiRunning and taste the potential it holds for you as a runner, and learned to deeply relax while feeling the technique in your body, it is time to play and experiment with all you've learned. It is what I do on every run. I play with directing the energy in my body and feeling the chi in ChiRunning doing its part. I play with what I've learned by experimenting, and carefully testing the limits of ChiRunning.

There are no limits. My T'ai Chi teacher, Master Xu, says there is infinite variety to our movement. Every time I run I'm always seeking the sweet spot, which, due to the nature of running, can change in an instant. We can learn to play in the infinitely variable world in which we run, be it a slight hill, a rough piece of pavement, or big mountain whose peak we must see.

Learning Program for Beginning Runners

Whether you're just starting to run or coming back from an injury or a long break from running, you'll probably feel a mixture of excitement, anxiety, and anticipation. Once you've decided to get in shape and reclaim your health, there is a real sense of purpose: "I'm going to do this. I'm going to get myself out there and run three or four times a week!" The sense that I get from many beginning runners is one of determination and purpose . . . combined with some fear.

Many of the fears that come up have familiar voices:

"I'm too out of shape. I get winded running down the block."
"Why the heck am I planning on running? Everyone knows you shouldn't run after you're 40. I'll ruin my knees."
"Running is just too hard."
"People who run all seem like fanatics."

But you're intrigued nonetheless. Maybe it's because you remember that great feeling you had when you used to run. Or maybe you're just looking for the quickest and easiest way to reclaim your health.

Well, you can put your fears to rest by knowing that for most people, running is a safe and effective way to get some great exercise at any age. Humans are meant to run. We're built for it. And when you learn to run with good, sound biomechanics combined with a sensible program, you can significantly reduce the possibility of hurting yourself. It doesn't have to be hard to get started, but it is wise to get started carefully and with a specific and manageable plan. As a new runner, you have the opportunity to learn good habits right from the start because you have what we affectionately call a "clean slate," with no bad habits. So, take your time. When you're running safely and efficiently, you'll be able to run joyfully for one mile or eventually 26 miles if you so desire. Here are some helpful hints.

- **Set aside twenty to thirty minutes every other day.** The best way to begin your program and get into a good habit with your fitness is to set aside twenty to thirty minutes every other day to get yourself started. Minutes are a better way to start than miles. This takes the comparative pressure off. Block out this time in your appointment calendar, just as you would for any other important event. Don't worry, you won't be running for the whole time at first, but you'll need at least that amount of time to do Body Looseners before you run and Stretches after (see Chapter 8, "Transitioning Into and Out of Running"). By practicing the ChiRunning form every other day, you will get a clear body memory of what you're learning.
- **Read the book, watch the DVD.** To get yourself comfortable with the concepts, I highly recommend reading at least through Chapter 5 along with viewing the ChiRunning DVD once through before you get started.
- **Take yourself through the ten lessons sequentially:** Repeat the lessons as many times as you would like. There is no time pressure.
- **Run slowly.** Begin running very slowly, taking very short strides. When you are first learning ChiRunning there is no reason to run fast. When practicing your technique, always run at a comfortable, conversational pace.
- **Run/walk.** The key for any beginner is to run only for as long as feels comfortable, whether it's thirty seconds or five minutes. If you feel you're out of breath or not focused, stop and walk for one minute. Then, check in with your posture alignment, reinstate whatever focus you are working on and begin running again. In ChiRunning, form comes first, so increase your distance for only as long as you can hold your form, then walk.
  - Run slow, walk fast. The best way to practice the ChiRunning *and* the ChiWalking focuses is to run slowly (1st or 2nd gear) but walk fast (65–75 strides/minute) during your walk breaks. This allows you to maintain a good sense of momentum even during the walk breaks.
  - If you can, try to maintain a 5:1 ratio of running to walking— five minutes of running followed by one minute of walking. As

you progress, you can increase the number of minutes running. Once you have built up to twenty to thirty minutes at a run/walk, you may be ready to just run, knowing you can always take a walking break if needed. Run regularly within your aerobic capacity, and within six to eight weeks your increase in aerobic conditioning will allow you to gradually phase out your walk breaks without feeling any extra strain.

- **Body Sense.** What is most important is that you get a feel in your body of what you should be doing. Take your time with each lesson until you have a strong Body Sense of the lesson.
- **Start a running journal or log.** In Chapter 6, "Program Development," we suggest you start a running journal or log and that you do a current assessment of your health and goals. It is a great idea to start that journal before getting started on these lessons.
- **Move on to pairs of focuses.** Once you've gotten through all the lessons, move on to working with the pairs of focuses at the end of this chapter. Create your own pairs that work for you.

See the ten lessons immediately following the next section.

Learning Program for Intermediate and Advanced Runners

If you're already a runner but new to learning the ChiRunning technique, this section is for you.

We start all runners the same way. Whether you're a total beginner or an elite competitor, we've found it much quicker and easier to teach you new movement habits rather than correcting your current habits. The main difference between this learning program and the one for beginning runners is that you will be learning the technique during your current running program. You have more running under your belt, so we start you with a program that doesn't include regular walk breaks. Here are some helpful ideas for you.

- **Take yourself through the ten lessons sequentially.** Go through the lessons at your own pace. Take your time; get a good feel for each focus and play with it. See how it feels in your running. If you feel you are already adept at any of the focuses, you may be able to combine some lessons.

- **Keep your current running program, but slow the pace.** Whatever your regular weekly running program is, don't change the amount of time you run. What we ask you to do is run for the same amount of time you're used to running, but commit to using that time to work on *form only*. Then, as you become skilled with the basic focuses, you can practice holding your form for longer and longer distances. As your body becomes increasingly conditioned to the ChiRunning technique, all you'll have to do is lean more, relax more . . . and speed happens.

  We recommend that form work always be done at a conversational aerobic pace . . . nothing faster. As long as you're running at a comfortable pace, you won't lose your aerobic conditioning. It's all about alignment and relaxation. Take the time up front to practice the focuses at a slower pace and learn to set up the conditions for speed to happen. Turn each practice run into a playful game of efficiency. As you become more efficient in your movement, you'll find that speed you're looking for, without the effort you're currently used to.

- **Take care of current injuries.** If you have any pains or injuries, work on correcting them first by applying the appropriate ChiRunning focuses. Leave any speed training drills out of your program until the injury goes away and until you've built up your aerobic capacity with your new technique. This will insure that your new running form is solid enough to support additional distance or speed without the risk of reinjury.

- **Rethink your race schedule.** We get letters all the time about how quickly ChiRunning has made a difference. It's great. However, it is best to really make sure you have the focuses in your body before racing. Consider rethinking your race schedule and getting your form up to speed first. Read more about speed and racing in Chapter 10.

- **Move on to pairs of focuses.** Once you've gotten through all the lessons, move on to working with the pairs of focuses at the end of this chapter. Create your own pairs that work for you.

- **Train smarter, not harder.** Although you'll be doing your workouts at a nice conversational aerobic pace, every run will require very precise focus and practice. Don't believe for a second that more physical effort is better. If you don't feel you're getting a good workout, you can always extend the length of your workouts to fit your needs.
- **Practice using your y'chi.** This is by far one of the single most important focuses to practice once you feel comfortable and familiar with all of the basic ChiRunning focuses (see Lesson Eight below).
- **Interval Form Focus training.** Review Chapter 6 and create a running program with a variety of types of runs. Make sure you include a Form Focus Run where you practice various Form Focuses in intervals (see page 152).

Ten Lessons for Learning the ChiRunning Technique

Whether you're a beginning runner or a seasoned runner, do the following progression of lessons sequentially. If you need more time with any given lesson, you can repeat the lesson in as many subsequent runs as you need to in order to get a clear Body Sense of what it should feel like. When you feel you have a clear sense of the lesson in your mind and body, move on to the next lesson. You could spend a week or more on any lesson.

LESSON ONE: GET STARTED IN A SIMPLE WAY BY PRACTICING POSTURE

Your first lesson is to practice and learn Posture all the way through the one-legged posture stance (pages 64–79). Take your time with this. Read and reread this section practicing each exercise. Don't skimp on learning posture. Using the DVD as a visual aid will be very helpful as well. All of this can be done in the comfort of your living room. Once you feel that you have a clear feeling of the one-legged posture stance in your body you're going to take it for a run.

When you're ready to try out your one-legged posture stance while running go to "How to Start Your Run" on page 115 and follow instructions 1–6. Don't worry about practicing the lean yet. Simply use your run to practice your one-legged posture stance. Do this for a couple of runs or until you feel comfortable feeling the one-legged stance while you're running. If you're a beginner do this in a walk/run mode and if you're an advanced runner practice the one-legged posture stance at a slow pace for one-minute intervals during one of your regular runs.

LESSON TWO: ENGAGE YOUR LEAN

- **Review the lean.** Review the section on leaning (pages 81–85) before heading out the door, then take it out for a "test drive."
- **Practice engaging your lean: The Three-step Process.**
  Step 1: While moving down the road, check in with your Column.
  Step 2: Drop your mental focus to the bottoms of your feet.
  Step 3: Keep your feet hitting where they are (at the bottom of your Column) and let your whole Column fall *slightly* in front of where your feet are hitting.

Balance yourself by practicing the Window of Lean Exercise (see page 84). Repeat the exercise three or four more times during every run. Practice adding the lean to your one-legged posture stance in this way for a week, or more if you need to.

When you engage and disengage the lean several times while maintaining your one-legged posture stance, you'll begin to feel the effect leaning has on your running. Over time, you will find your comfort zone with your lean, so play with it. If you begin to feel any tension in your calves or shins, it means you're leaning too far forward and holding your lean by tightening your lower leg muscles. Back off a bit and try to balance yourself in the "window of lean"—not too far forward, and not too upright. This is subtle stuff. You don't need to lean as much as you think.

LESSON THREE: PICK UP YOUR HEELS

In Lesson 2 you practiced leaning to engage the pull of gravity. In this lesson you'll practice picking up your heels, and learn how to *not* push off with your toes as you fall forward. You will be lifting your ankles and peeling your heels off the ground, first in a standing position, then walking, and then at a slow jogging pace.

- **Review Passive Lower Leg:** (pages 87–88).
- **Do the Pick Up Your Heels exercise:** (page 87) Practice for a few minutes.
- **Do the Walk with Peeling Up the Foot Exercise:** (page 88) Walk for five to ten minutes alternating between picking up your feet and walking how you normally do, to feel the difference in lower leg usage.
- **Begin running as in Lesson 1**
- **Pretend you have *no lower legs:*** Do this in one-minute intervals with one-minute breaks between. Focus on peeling your heels up with each step. You can also use the visualizations on page 96 "The Wheel." During your one-minute breaks, keep running, but let your lower legs go as limp as you can.

LESSON FOUR: THE SAND PIT EXERCISE

In this lesson, you'll continue to practice relaxing your lower legs and picking up your feet by doing the Sand Pit Exercise a number of times before running. A track is best for this exercise, because you'll be alternating running over sand with running on a firm surface.

- **Review Sand Pit Exercise** (pages 89–90). Go back and forth over the sand pit until you can leave clean, crisp footprints with both feet. Check carefully for foot splay-out, heel strike, or craters from toeing off. Spend at least fifteen minutes crossing the sand pit, clearing your prints when necessary.
- **Sand pit/track workout.** Run across the sand pit followed immediately (without stopping) by one lap around the track. Repeat four times, or more if necessary. Do this exercise anytime you feel tension in your lower legs.

LESSON FIVE: PELVIC ROTATION

The next thing to practice, after picking up your feet and relaxing your lower legs, is pelvic rotation. In this lesson you'll practice pelvic rotation and learn how to have a smooth, relaxed stride.

- **Review pelvic rotation** (pages 97–100).
- **Review the Pool Running Drill** (page 100).
- **Do the Pool Running Drill.** Find a level place to run and repeat the last step in the drill until you can clearly feel your pelvis rotating while you run. Don't force anything. Remember, you're not trying to *do* anything. Just watch for, and allow your pelvis to rotate. Keeping your pelvis level is essential.

LESSON SIX: SWING YOUR LEGS TO THE REAR

This lesson brings together Lessons Two and Five, leaning and rotating your pelvis to produce a rearward leg swing. As your Column falls forward, your pelvis rotates, allowing your legs to swing out the back.

- **Review Swing Your Legs to the Rear** (page 91).
- **Practice the Pool Running exercise.** Use the Pool Running exercise as a warm-up.
- **Practice One-legged posture while running.** Run for five minutes at a slow pace just practicing your one-legged posture stances.
- **Focus your attention on T12/L1** (page 99). With your focus on the Pivot Point, feel your entire lower body rotate with each stride. Every time each leg swings to the rear, *let your hip go with it.*
- **Feel your feet and legs swinging rearward as soon as your foot hits the ground.** This is impossible to do without leaning.

LESSON SEVEN: ARM SWING, HEAD, NECK, AND SHOULDERS

As you learn to let your lower body swing with each stride, it is important to stabilize your upper body so that your lower body can move more freely and easily. In this lesson, you'll learn how to swing your arms to stabilize your shoulders, thus allowing your lower body its full range of motion.

- **Review and practice the Arm Swing** (page 102). Pay close attention to hand, elbow, and shoulder positions.
- **Combine Pelvic Rotation and Arm Swing.** After running for ten minutes, focusing only on your arm swing, add in the Pelvic Rotation and feel your legs swing to the rear with each stride. Run for ten more minutes feeling your legs *and* your elbows swing rearward with your shoulders always facing forward.
- **Add in your lean.** During the last ten minutes of your workout, practice feeling your arms and legs swinging out behind you while your Column leans (falls) forward. Feel your Column falling forward balancing out the movement of your arms and legs swinging rearward. Practicing in this way will help you find the "window of lean" more easily.

LESSON EIGHT: Y'CHI AND THE KNEE-BENDING EXERCISE

This exercise is designed to give you a clear sense of running without pushing off with your feet.

- **Review the Knee-Bending Exercise** (pages 92–94) **and review y'chi** (page 85). Find a quiet, flat open stretch of road or track. Do a warm-up run for ten minutes and then go through four repeats of the Knee-Bending Exercise. Be sure to closely follow the instructions and do all three steps for each repeat.
- **Practice your y'chi.** Before you do the third step, while standing in place, focus your eyes on some spot or object in the distance and don't break your gaze from the time you begin moving forward until you stop. Allow your visual connection with your "goal" to pull your body forward while you're moving through all the steps of the Knee-Bending Exercise.
- **Continue running.** After doing the Knee-Bending Exercise, run at a comfortable pace with your countdown timer set to repeat every two minutes. When your beeper goes off, stop and do the Knee-

Bending Exercise, going through all three steps. Then, relax back into a comfortable pace until your watch beeps again. Repeat this exercise until the end of your workout. Cool down.

LESSON NINE: CADENCE AND METRONOME

In this lesson you'll be practicing to run with a steady cadence by running with a metronome. If you don't have one, we highly recommend you get one, as it is the best way I've ever found to learn to change your stride length. We have them available at ChiRunning.com.

- **Review the Metronome** (page 112).
- **Find your current cadence.** Do your warm-up run for ten minutes and then, while running at a comfortable steady pace, count the number of steps your right foot takes in one minute. That's your current cadence.
- **Set your metronome** to the number of strides/minute you are currently running and match your cadence to your metronome for the rest of your run.
- **Vary your speed.** Practice running at various speeds while always matching your cadence to the metronome. Give yourself the whole range of speeds, from very slow to fast. Try to not miss a single beat! You'll find that it forces you to lengthen or shorten your stride depending on what speed you're running.
- **Increase your cadence.** If your current cadence is slower than 85 strides/minute, increase your cadence by one step/minute each week until you reach 85. (Shorter runners should aim for running closer to 90 spm; taller, overweight, or older runners should aim for a minimum of 85 spm.)

LESSON TEN: GEARS AND STRIDE LENGTH

In this last lesson you'll use your metronome *and* your countdown timer to practice lengthening and shortening your stride to increase your efficiency. You'll also learn to lean more or lean less in order to change your speed. Before starting this workout, set your countdown timer to beep at one-minute intervals and set your metronome to your current cadence. This is a great lesson to go back to and repeat often.

Laying the groundwork for a future of highly efficient running is a continual but highly fruitful process.

- **Review "Gears, Cadence, and Stride Length"** (pages 106–112).
- **Run in first gear (warm-up pace).** Start your metronome and warm up for five minutes at your current cadence with 1 inch of lean (first gear).
- **Run in second gear (training pace).** Start your countdown timer and "shift" to second gear by adding 1 more inch of lean. Remember to use the three-step method of engaging your lean (see Lesson Two). When your countdown timer beeps, let off your lean and return to first gear for the next minute. For ten minutes, alternate between first and second gear every minute.
- **Run in third gear (race pace).** For the next ten minutes alternate between second and third gears. Always relax more and let your stride open up whenever you increase your lean. Shorten your stride whenever you let off your "gas pedal."
- **Play with your gears.** For the remainder of your run, just play with adding or subtracting to your lean in 1-inch increments while adjusting your stride length accordingly—all the time staying with the beat of your metronome.

LIFE AFTER THE LESSONS

By the time you've worked your way through all ten lessons, you will have a very clear grasp on all of the various aspects of the basic ChiRunning form. To help you in your continuing practice of mastering your body and the Form Focuses, here's a list of pairs of focuses to work with on future runs. For convenience, the pairs of focuses are listed by body area, but feel free to work with them in any order that suits your interest or running needs. You can do them in one of two ways:

Workout A: Do the first focus of the pair for the first third of your run and then do the second focus for the second third. For the final third combine both focuses.

Workout B: If you use a countdown timer, you can alternate single focuses for one-minute intervals for two-thirds of your run and finish doing both focuses.

When you get to where you feel confident with the pairs of focuses, you can challenge yourself and practice doing two pairs of focuses during your runs. Use the same format as explained in workouts A and B by alternating *pairs* of focuses just as you did with the single focuses.

At some point in your process of mastery, some of these focuses will be so integrated into your mind and body that they'll become second nature and you'll only have to directly work on the focuses you haven't fully learned. Eventually your ChiRunning practice will become an intuitive way of running. That being said, there is one focus I *always* have to remember to engage: leveling my pelvis, which keeps me in the present moment and my core engaged.

CHIRUNNING FOCUSES IN PAIRS

Posture

One-legged posture stance/Bend opposite knee
Lengthen back of neck/Level pelvis
Feel your Column/Feel a midfoot strike
Connect the dots/relax everything else

Lean

Shoulders forward/Elbows back
Upper body forward/Lower body rearward
Hold the "C" shape/Balance in the "window of lean"
Level your pelvis/Lean from your ankles

Lower Body

Focus on the Pivot Point/Rotate lower body below T12/L1
Midfoot strike/Let your hip swing back with leg
Circular feet: Peel heels up over opposite ankle/Knees down
Knee bending/One-legged posture stance

Pelvic Rotation

Rotate your pelvis/Feel yourself run level to the ground

Small rotation at slower speeds/Large rotation at faster speeds

Level pelvis/Rotate pelvis from T12/L1

Upper Body

Shoulders squared forward/Elbows back

Y'chi focused forward/Elbows back

Lengthen back of neck/Open your chest

Forward lean with Column/Elbows and legs swinging rearward

Lengthen back of neck/Focus your y'chi ahead

Cadence and Breathing

Level pelvis/Belly breathing (inhale through nose, exhale through mouth)

Match your breath rate to your cadence: 3:2 or 2:1 out/in

Gears and Stride Length

Increase lean/Lengthen stride

Decrease lean/Shorten stride

Sustain each gear for one minute/Relax lower legs

Steady cadence (metronome)/Cycle up and down through gears

Body Sensing and Relaxation

Level your pelvis/Relax your lower back

Rotate your pelvis/Relax your lower back

Relax your shoulders/Lengthen your neck

Level your pelvis/Rotate your pelvis

Relax lower legs/"C" shape

Relax your wrists/Relax your ankles

Level your pelvis/Relax your glutes

CHAPTER SIX

Program Development

We are what we repeatedly do. Excellence, then, is not an act, but a habit. —ARISTOTLE

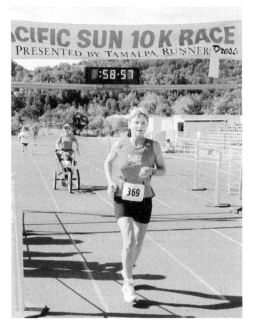

Figure 62—Nancy Weninger, age 55, triathlete and ChiRunning student

P rogram development adds the ingredient of *duration* to your Form Focuses. Whether it's measured in minutes for a beginner or in hours for a marathoner, a part of the process of learning the ChiRunning technique is integrating the Form Focuses into your running for longer periods of time. This is where having a well-planned running program will guarantee safe and successful development, one based on the core principles of ChiRunning.

THE FORMULA FOR SUCCESS

The formula for developing a successful ChiRunning program is *form, distance, and speed*—in that specific order. This three-stage method will guarantee that your program will build safely and gradually because you won't fall prey to the power running mind-set of "no pain, no gain" and get injured by overtraining.

Work on your *form* before anything else. As you are able to hold that together for longer periods of time, you will be building core strength while becoming more relaxed. Together, these components create the foundation for increased *distance*. When you can hold your form together for a longer period of time, increased *speed* with a lower perceived exertion level becomes attainable because you're combining efficient running form with a good distance base. But if you bypass efficiency and distance for speed, you might encounter an injury or a setback in your running program.

There are about as many types of training programs as there are runners. All of them profess to be the best training program available to get you faster, or into great shape, or to the other end of a marathon. A training formula is like a recipe for cookies—if you follow the directions, you'll end up with cookies. But if ten people follow the same recipe, they'll end up with ten different batches of cookies. In the end, recipes are really only general guidelines.

Instead, I'm going to offer you some valuable guidelines for approaching a training program. You will be an active participant, assessing your current state and designing a program that suits your specific needs.

FORM, DISTANCE, AND SPEED:
THE THREE DEVELOPMENT STAGES OF
THE CHIRUNNING TECHNIQUE

FORM: OPENNESS TO CHANGE

As you begin to set up your ChiRunning program, most of the early emphasis should be directed toward form work. If you're a beginning runner, start off by working mostly on your form and then slowly add distance. If you're a seasoned runner, it's wise to give yourself a couple of months to hone in on your form and lighten up on specific pacing or race goals. Trust me, the sacrifice is worth it.

Here's my favorite story about working on form for long-term improvement. I will paraphrase an article that appeared in the August 14, 2000, issue of *Time* magazine. In 1997 Tiger Woods was at the top of the heap, winning the British Open, the U.S. Open, the PGA Championship, and the Masters, all at the ripe old age of 20. But after watching endless videos of himself, he came to the conclusion that although he was winning a lot of tournaments, his swing needed some pretty deep reworking. In his words, "My swing really sucks."

His coach told him that he could do it, but not to expect to win any golf tournaments for a while. Tiger was willing to take that risk because he knew it was the only way he could realize long-term improvement.

As he spent the next nineteen months working on his swing, Tiger won only one tour event out of nineteen starts. The press was writing him off as a flash in the pan, and fans became increasingly disappointed.

Then, one day in May 1999, when Tiger was preparing for the Byron Nelson Classic, he finally felt something happen in his swing. It was exactly what he'd been looking for, and the rest, as they say, is history. He then proceeded to win ten of the next fourteen events, going on to win the prestigious Grand Slam of golf at the age of twenty-four.

He did it all by first taking a good long look at his form, establishing the goal of improving his swing, and then meticulously doing everything in his power, physically and mentally, to improve his form. The two ChiRunning principles that stand out here are Gradual Progress (making small continuous improvements) and Non-identification (not being afraid of what others will think). Since then, Tiger has reconstructed his swing from scratch several more times.

If Tiger Woods is willing to make a form change, putting his career at risk, you might be willing to slow down your pace—maybe skip that upcoming race and get into working toward the long-term results that will keep you running well for a lifetime.

DISTANCE: INSTATING NEW HABITS

Many people have a particular distance in mind that they would like to accomplish. I respect that desire, because I have it too. But as you might guess, the *distance* I'm talking about is concerned more with the means than the end. I like to talk about distance as a tool to deepen your knowledge of the focuses and your own body. Once again, the path becomes the goal.

In ChiRunning, distance is the means by which you instate new healthy habits into your running. It is by repeating and holding the Form Focuses over time and distance that they'll become ingrained in your running technique.

The true test of ChiRunning is in how long you can hold your running form. It's about quality, not quantity. Your mind and body work best as a team. Your mind, directing the show, introduces the new habit, while your body, through long-term constant repetition, learns to form a new "groove" in which to operate. Once you begin to feel the correct motion, it will soon become a habit, and then it's *yours*. It is the workings of the mind that are being tested over long distances.

The first step is to teach your mind to be as focused as possible, so it can direct your body. In practicing a new Form Focus, your mind will naturally go through periods of remembering the focus and then being distracted. When your mind becomes distracted—and it *will*—it'll stay distracted until you bring your focus back into play. Use a watch with a ten-minute countdown timer as a reminder to go back to your focus. Every time you catch yourself being distracted, just bring your attention back to the focus, make the necessary physical adjustments, and continue with your run. Each time you return to your focus, renew your intention to hold it. Repetitive reminders from your mind will train your body to hold a focus longer. This is not any different from how a meditation instructor would teach you to meditate. If you're sitting and observing your breath, *that's* your focus; whenever you find your mind wandering, you drop what you're thinking about and return to your breath. ChiRunning is like doing a running meditation. As you learn to hold each ChiRunning focus for a longer distance, you'll be able to add in a second focus, and then a third, until eventually you can run with many happening simultaneously.

SPEED: THE ICING ON THE CAKE

As much as I downplay the need for speed, running all out is one of my favorite things to do. It's exhilarating and fun. When you have your form together and your body is comfortable with running, all of the training comes together and speed happens. Here is a letter from a client who expresses his delight with running fast and its apparent ease.

This letter is from a person who wrote to me after only one hourlong session of coaching.

Dear Danny,

My introduction to ChiRunning was nothing less than life-changing. It makes so much sense, and for someone who loves to run as much as I do, it affords me the real vision of being able to run for the rest of my life, injury-free.

Not only does ChiRunning excite me with its potential to avoid injuries, but since our time together, I've been playing with it and been amazed at the results. When I normally complete a run, my calves and quads are tight, and I can really feel them as I stretch. Now I barely notice the muscles and any soreness. There is even an energizing afterward.

What really surprised me was the improvement in my time and distance. What used to be a relaxed 8-minute-pace daily run has turned into a 6:50-to-7-minute pace. Mind-blowing!! Today I played with it at the track and paced myself at 6:50/mile pace without much more of an effort than I used to put out running the old way.

Chris

Speed comes last in the progression of form, distance, and speed because it is totally dependent on the quality of its two predecessors, form and distance. Speed is the by-product of your ability to do the necessary focuses in the right proportion. In the end, your technique will support your speed.

In ChiRunning, speed doesn't come from pushing; it comes from an increased ability to focus and relax; it should not be the solitary goal of any workout. Running faster can be fun, especially when it is the by-product of a well-done process.

CREATING A RUNNING PROGRAM

Going on vacation, for me, is a sacred event. It doesn't happen that often, so it's crucial that I spend much of my vacation time enjoying myself. Vacations are the best metaphor I can think of to introduce the concept of planning ahead, because most people have some experience with them, and the subject usually brings up lots of emotions.

How would you plan your vacation with a minimum of glitches? You might want to think back to some of your more memorable hassles and plan to avoid repeating the same experiences—like the time you booked a week in the tropics at a bargain price only to realize when you got there that it was their monsoon season, or the time you weren't aware there would be a Hell's Angels convention at your campground during the week of your stay. Maybe you've learned that having a full day at home before going back to work has made all the difference.

Like planning a perfect vacation, this section is devoted to helping you design a running program that really works for you—on all levels, because it is grounded in *your* experience.

Building a good program should take into account:

1. Your present condition
2. Your aspirations
3. The demands of your current life
4. The specifics of each run

By following these four steps you will be able to develop a well-planned, well-rounded program that will be organized, sequential, and in tune with your body's needs and capabilities.

Set yourself up with a running journal and take notes on your answers. A journal can serve multiple functions.

- You'll have a record of where you started from. It's great to look back to your beginnings and acknowledge the changes you've made.
- You'll learn over time what works and what doesn't work, and what to focus on if you have a repeating issue.
- The process of writing gets you in touch with and affirms what you really want.

We have logs available on the ChiRunning website.

ASSESS YOUR CURRENT STATE

It is important to begin with an honest personal assessment of where you're beginning, so there are no illusions about what you can and can't do relative to your running. In other words, start from where you're at, not from somewhere else. Nobody likes to encounter the old one-step-forward-three-steps-back scenario. You can come up with a great running program, but if your present state isn't taken into account, it could end up being too ambitious, too time-consuming, or beyond your current capabilities in some way.

There are three parts to the assessment process: physical, mental, and your ability with the ChiRunning skills.

The Physical Assessment

Here are some questions to ask yourself as you sit down to design your program. Remember, this is for your eyes only, so be as honest as you can.

- Are you currently nursing any injuries, aches, or pains?
- Do you have any physical conditions that would warrant a doctor's approval or consultation before beginning a running program?
- What is the maximum number of miles or minutes you could comfortably run today?
- Are you overweight? Do you use running for weight management?

Also, it's a good idea to know your resting heart rate (RHR) and check it once a month or so. Here's how to find your RHR. Before you go to bed, lay your watch next to you within easy reach from where you're sleeping. When you wake up in the morning, before you do anything else, reach for your watch and take your pulse by holding your pointer and middle fingers on your neck, just next to your throat beneath your lower jaw, while holding your watch in the other hand so you can read it. Count the number of heartbeats in fifteen seconds and then multiply that number by four to get beats per minute. Jot it down in your running or walking log for future reference. Those of you who are starting off in the lower end of the fitness spectrum will get to enjoy the largest drop in this number as you work out more frequently, so you have a lot to look forward to.

The Mental Assessment: Thinking/Feeling

Ponder some of the following questions and see what pops up in your head. Getting a clear sense of your thoughts and feelings regarding your program will allow you to tailor a running program to fit your specific needs.

- How much of a part of your life do you want running to occupy?
- Why do you run?
- What do you want from running?
- Do you feel better training with a group? Alone? With a partner?
- How good are you at being self-motivated, with staying on a training program?
- Would you like to achieve a certain distance or pace?
- Is there a specific race you'd like to train for?
- What are your fears around running?

Assess Your ChiRunning Skills

Once you've read Chapter 4 and worked through the ten lessons in Chapter 5, then evaluate your strengths and weaknesses with the ChiRunning technique. For example, leaning might come naturally to you, but relaxing might not. The evaluation is best done immediately after each run, and should be a regular practice. Get out your running journal and write down any visualizations or reminders that worked particularly well, along with areas where you experienced some difficulty. In this way you'll be consistently assessing your current ChiRunning skills and working on new ones. I always have at least one area of focus that I pay attention to during any given run.

Questions to Ask Yourself

Which Form Focuses are the hardest for me to do?

What are the weak areas of my ChiRunning technique?

Do I clearly understand the instructions for each focus?

The answers to these questions will provide you with a clearer view of what to work on during your run.

Later in this chapter I will describe various types of workouts and list the specific focuses that best match the workout. If you find yourself slow to pick up one of the focuses, I suggest doing a run that accentuates it. The body learns best through repetition, which shortens the time it takes to learn the focus.

SET BODY-ORIENTED GOALS

Now that you have assessed your current state, you can readily determine some legitimate goals that will truly serve your best interests. By "legitimate" I mean goals that have a depth of thinking and feeling behind them—and which won't throw off the balance of your life.

There is definitely something to be said for setting goals, but be careful that they don't slip into being results-oriented. That internal conversation might sound something like, "I want to run faster than my neighbor," or "I want to win that race." By contrast, a body-oriented goal would be one that wells up from inside. The goal should also be within your capacity to manifest in a healthy way, given the right conditions and a realistic time frame. There's nothing wrong with a goal if you're listening to your body and asking it a reasonable request.

A results-oriented goal might sound like "I want to run a 6-minute mile." Translated into a body-oriented goal, it would sound more like "I want to be a faster runner." The former statement holds me to a specific path that will be considered successful only if I run a 6-minute mile. If a 6:23 mile is the fastest I'll ever run, I'll never be totally happy, because I never reached my goal.

On the other hand, the goal of being a faster runner automatically puts the emphasis on the *process,* because being faster is a relative statement. Faster than what? Faster than who? Faster than I am now? Stating that I want to be faster directs my attention to what my *body* will have to go through to achieve that goal. This is how the emphasis is taken off the goal and put onto the process. It's great to have the goal of running a 5K, a 10K, or a marathon, but be sure to allow yourself enough training time to really enjoy the process and get something of value from it.

Think of any goals that you'd like to achieve, and write them down in your running journal. If you sense that there are any results-oriented goals popping up in the list, just move them to a separate list . . . for later disposal. Here are some more suggestions for body-oriented goals: ease of movement, fluidity, no injuries, injury recovery, increased fitness level, improved diet, feeling good about yourself, getting outdoors.

Here are a few of the ones I've worked on with success over the years:
- To run with no knee pain
- To finish a marathon with no recovery time needed
- To run without injury
- To finish my runs feeling better than when I started

SCHEDULING YOUR PROGRAM

Now that you've done your homework of assessment and goal setting, it's time to put it all together into a workable schedule. You'll need to get out your running journal and your calendar. The basic idea is to come up with a workout schedule that won't throw the rest of your life out of balance. I mean, who needs a life that's more difficult? Whether you're starting a new running program or adding running to an established fitness program, these questions will guide you through the process of carving out the time. If you already have a running program, the questions will help you refine it.

In your running journal write down your answers to the following questions.

1. How many days a week do you want to run? (I recommend at least three but no more than six days a week, if running is your main form of exercise. It's easier to keep a momentum going with your workouts if they're not too spread out and if you're not running all the time.)
2. Given that number of days, which specific days of the week work best to support it?
3. On each of those chosen days, how many minutes could you dedicate to a workout? Be sure to include any travel time and transition times, along with your actual running time. Don't crunch your time if you can help it.
4. On each of those chosen days, what time would you be most likely to guarantee a workout would happen?

Go immediately to your calendar and block out these times.

These questions require you to take into account what is happening in the rest of your life, especially around the time when your run is scheduled to happen. This requires that you hold yourself responsible to do what you say you're going to do. These steps are the backbone of a consistent running program. The whole idea is to develop a successful plan that blends seamlessly with the rest of your life.

Treat your workouts as appointments. If someone calls you asking to get together during one of these blocks of time, just say that you have something scheduled and ask if there's another time you could meet.

THE WELL-ROUNDED RUNNING PROGRAM

A well-rounded running program is one that will condition your body, build core strength, improve your circulation, increase your range of motion, increase your aerobic capacity, strengthen your heart, help to relieve stress, and generally improve your physical, mental, and spiritual well-being. The chart on the next page shows three sample running programs. Level I is for beginners and those coming back from injury who want to build a solid base in their conditioning and running technique. Level II is for intermediate runners who are looking to improve their conditioning base and reduce their PRE. Level III is for seasoned runners and competitors wanting to improve their conditioning base, maximize their efficiency, and increase their speed.

There are five types of runs that will cover the whole spectrum of training situations. Even though you will be practicing many of the ChiRunning focuses on each run, certain focuses are particularly suited to certain runs. Each run will have a unique set of characteristics that contribute to the whole of your technique. When the ChiRunning focuses become an integral part of your running, you will have a built-in set of tools to use in any situation.

Full descriptions of each of the listed runs immediately follow the chart.

Sample Running Programs

Day	Level I	Level II	Level III
1	Off	Speed intervals or form intervals	Speed intervals
2	Fun run or form intervals	Hill run	Hill run
3	Off	Off	Tempo run
4	Fun run or form intervals	Tempo run	Off
5	Off	Off	Fun run or form intervals
6	Fun run or form intervals	Long run	Long run
7	Off or fun run	Off	Off

INTERVALS: FORM AND SPEED

I recommend two types of intervals: form intervals and speed intervals. The form intervals are a great way to practice and learn various form focuses during timed intervals. The speed intervals are meant for intermediate ChiRunners who've practiced and learned the ChiRunning technique and are conditioning themselves for an upcoming race.

Form Intervals

I highly recommend this workout for beginning runners or for those coming back after a long break. This is a fun workout. In fact, you can always substitute this run for a scheduled fun run. For the duration of your run, you will alternate between focusing and not focusing—one minute on, one minute off, one minute on, one minute off, until you finish. Before your run, go over your list of focuses that you feel a need to work on.

- If you have a sports watch with a repeat countdown timer, set it to beep every minute. Focus on one aspect of your technique for a minute, then relax and don't focus for a minute.
- Once you're warmed up and running at a comfortable pace, start your countdown timer. When the beep goes off, bring all of your attention to the focus that you picked and do everything in your power to hold it for the entire minute *without a single lapse in concentration.* It's only a minute, so try hard to stay with it. When you hear the next beep, drop the focus, relax, and enjoy yourself for a minute.
- When the beep goes off again, go back to concentrating on your specific focus for the next minute.
- Repeat this pattern of alternating focus with relaxation for the rest of your run.
- If you've picked two focuses, do one of them for the first third of your run, and do the second one for the second third. In the final third, try to hold both focuses at the same time for one-minute intervals.

For beginners, this is one of the most efficient ways to learn the individual focuses, because in a thirty-minute run, you'll practice engaging a specific focus fifteen times!

The three focuses that I recommend starting with are:

1. Holding your posture straight
2. Leaning from your feet
3. Picking up your feet as you run

Speed Intervals

This workout is a favorite because it's really fun. It's an exercise in instant gratification, because I'm not *trying* to run faster. I'm trying to hold all of my Form Focuses together, then using my times as a confirmation. Speed is *not* the primary goal of this workout. There are so many other things that are more important to work on that thinking of speed would only serve as a distraction. The simple definition of "interval" is a period of highly focused running followed by a brief recovery period at a restful pace.

Speed is a by-product of proper form. So a speed interval is really just another type of form interval in which you set up the right conditions for speed to happen. No matter what level of runner you are, speed intervals should be undertaken only when you feel comfortable with holding the focuses. It is a prime opportunity to practice the principle of Gradual Progress because you're always working from slow to fast, from small to big.

If you would like to increase your basic running speed, pick one day each week to go to your local track and do some 400-meter intervals (400 meters is one lap around most tracks). Focus on one or more of the focuses below for a lap, then rest for a lap. Repeat this sequence four to ten times, depending on your level of conditioning. If you don't know how many intervals you should do, let your body tell you. Start off with four and then Body Sense whether or not you can handle more. Listen carefully to your body, and you'll know when you're done.

Follow the Gradual Progress rule and run your first interval the slowest. It's tempting to take off fast on the first one, since you usually feel fresh at the beginning of a workout. Don't be tempted. People often start off with a fast first interval, then get a little slower with each successive one until the last one, in which they barely hang on to any semblance of form. Additionally, they start each interval as fast as they can, burning out most of their energy during the first half of the lap and struggle to keep the same speed at the finish. So be sure to start slow enough not to exhaust all your energy at the outset.

You'll get a much better workout by letting each interval be a loosening exercise for the next one. As your workout progresses, every additional interval will be a little faster, not because you're pushing harder but because your joints and muscles are looser and more relaxed.

When you've done your last interval, jog a couple of easy laps and congratulate yourself on a job well done.

Here are the key focuses to work on during your speed intervals.

- Start off slowly, and *very* gradually increase your lean throughout the length of the interval.
- Relax your lower body (hips, pelvis, and legs) as you lean more.
- Allow your stride to lengthen behind you as you increase your lean.
- Maintain a steady cadence at all times (85 to 90 strides per minute each leg).
- Engage your upper body more at higher speeds. Keep your shoulders relaxed and your elbows swinging fully out the back.
- Relax your lower back as you run faster. Let your abdominals hold your lean in place.
- Use your core muscles more and your legs less.
- Pick up your feet higher, but keep your knees low as you increase your lean. Don't pick up your knees, or you'll be using unnecessary effort.

LONG, SLOW DISTANCE RUN

I look forward to doing the LSD run each week—it's like looking forward to hanging out with an old friend. It's pure enjoyment! If my week has been particularly stressful, I can head into the woods knowing that I'll be a different person when I arrive back at my car. It's that predictable. It's a time for me, a time to let the dust settle and gather my thoughts, watch the seasons change, or just explore new territory. I'm not concerned about speed or distance; it's just time on my feet that I'm looking for.

The long run is a perfect opportunity to spend lots of time working on your focuses. I would say that relaxing is the most important thing to focus on. Do a Body Scan (see Chapter 3) every ten minutes, and watch for any place in your body that feels tense or tight. Then focus on relaxing that particular area. If you can hold the focus of relaxing for the entire run, you will finish your run feeling like you just got a great massage. This level of relaxation can be brought into all of your runs. Other focuses to practice on your long run are cadence, and posture, but not speed.

Because this run is done at a relaxed pace it does wonders for building your aerobic capacity by triggering your body to produce more extensive capillary beds. As your muscles improve oxygen uptake, all your runs will go better, because more of the oxygen from your lungs gets to your muscles, creating better efficiency. For those of you who want to be faster, the long run is what gives you the aerobic base to apply to speed training later on.

How long should a long run be? As long as you want, given the current capacity of your body and whatever amount of time you can afford. How much time would you like? If you're a beginning runner, your long run might be thirty minutes. When I was training to run the Leadville Trail 100-Mile Endurance Run, my long run was 40 miles every Sunday. That earned me permanent status in the lunatic-fringe category of runners. Now two hours once a week, year round, feels just fine. Your long run should not be so long that it leaves you wiped out. You should end this run feeling pleasantly tired.

FUN RUN

A fun run is just what it sounds like. When you've had a tough day or a sleepless night, or when you notice that you've been taking yourself way too seriously lately, it's time to go for a fun run. It can also be used as a recovery run following a long run or a fast run.

Go explore a new area. Go window-shopping. Go to a beautiful nature spot. Take a friend on a tour of your favorite running route. Leave your watch at home, and don't think about pace or distance. The emphasis of the run is on letting yourself relax physically and mentally. Don't take anything seriously (especially yourself); just have fun.

HILL RUN

A hill run can be of any intensity, from mellow, rolling country roads to steep trails. Use your best judgment. If you've never run hills and would like to, find easy ones to start with and run up only as far as is comfortable, then turn around and come back down. Like speed workouts, hills shouldn't be done until you get familiar and comfortable with holding the basic ChiRunning Form Focuses. If you run hills too early on when you're learning ChiRunning, your body could default to the way you used to run hills, thus complicating and lengthening the learning process. Since running up and down hills is a skill unto itself, I have given a full explanation of hill-running techniques in Chapter 7.

TEMPO RUN

A tempo run is the only run in this series of workouts that builds in both distance and speed. Seasoned runners use it for race practice. The distance is generally 4 to 8 miles, depending on your conditioning level. I don't recommend this workout for beginning runners or for anyone who doesn't have a good working knowledge of the ChiRunning focuses.

The object is to start off at a comfortable pace and slowly increase your lean over the length of the run. It might feel a bit faster than you're used to, because you're trying to do negative splits: each mile gets progressively faster, so your mile split times get smaller. If you're training for a race and you want to average an 8:52 pace, you would start off running slower than your average pace and end the run going faster than your average pace (as shown below).

Mile 1: 9:00
Mile 2: 8:55
Mile 3: 8:50
Mile 4: 8:45

Your average pace for the 4 miles would be 8:52. You can adjust these numbers to fit your own training needs. The most difficult part of the workout is doing the math.

A tempo run is a lesson in technique, not strength. The goal is to feel the *same* perceived effort level and the *same* cadence throughout even though your speed increases with each mile.

"You're nuts! How can that be possible?" you might say.

Well, I won't argue with you about whether or not I'm nuts. But it is entirely possible to do this workout as I've proposed. It's a matter of slowly increasing your lean while relaxing your body, and that's it in a nutshell.

Here's how the concept works. In ChiRunning, the more you lean the more your stride opens up behind you, not in front of you. The best way to lengthen your stride is to relax from your Pivot Point, which in turn allows your legs to swing more freely from your hips.

Keep your cadence uniform by using a metronome. This isn't just a recommendation; it's a requirement if you really want to learn to lengthen your stride. I set mine for 90 beats per minute and start it up as soon as I take my first step into my run. If you're used to running with a slower cadence, set the metronome for a minimum of 85 beats per minute. The best place to do this run is on a track. That way you can pace yourself by checking your timer every lap.

If you've never done a run like this and you don't know what pace you should run, let your body tell you. Jog a couple of warm-up laps at a very easy pace, do your Body Looseners, and then start your run at a comfortable second gear pace. If you have a stopwatch that records split times, hit the split button after each lap. The next lap should be one second faster. That's not a lot. Subsequently each lap will be a second faster until you've done the last lap. After 4 miles you will have run sixteen laps, so your last lap should be sixteen seconds faster than the first.

This is a *very* slow rate of increase in speed, so watch the timer closely. If you run the first lap in 2:00 minutes and the second lap in 1:55, you can let off on the gas pedal a little in the next lap. This is one of the best Body Sensing exercises, because you have to listen closely to your body and make tiny adjustments in speed. Nothing drastic here. It's one of my favorite runs, because I like the challenge of seeing how close I can come to the target time for each lap. If I come across the lap marker at 1:45, I know on the next lap I'll be looking for 1:44 to show up on the watch. It's fun, in a different kind of way, and very challenging.

To change your speed, you will be using your lean, not your leg strength. If you do a run like this once a week, you'll be a master at

The Five Workouts and Their Relative Areas of Focus

TYPE OF RUN	1 TEMPO RUN	2 HILL RUN	3 INTERVAL RUN	4 LONG RUN	5 FUN RUN OR RECOVERY RUN
AREA OF FOCUS					
Posture	X	X		X	X
Lean	X		X	X	
Cadence	X	X		X	X
Gears	X	X	X		
Arm swing	X	X	X		
Hip swing	X	X		X	X
Core strength	X	X	X		
Aerobic capacity				X	X
Cardiovascular		X	X		

pacing in no time, which will be a huge advantage in races. Everyone in your pace group will shoot away from the start line, and you'll be a little ways back in the pack, smiling, knowing that you will pass them all later.

THE FIVE WORKOUTS
AND THEIR RELATIVE FOCUSES

Since each of the five types of runs offers its own benefits to your overall ChiRunning technique, on the previous page is a table showing which Form Focuses are best learned in each of the five workouts.

CROSS-TRAINING FOR RUNNING

People often ask me if they should do any cross-training for their running. If your goal is to improve your running, you can be practicing your ChiRunning skills all day long. I highly recommend ChiWalking for runners. If you think about leveling your pelvis and relaxing your lower legs during your non-running hours on your feet, you'll be practicing good movement skills with every step. I recommend practicing your posture all day long, whether you're sitting at your desk, driving your car, or carrying groceries. I believe in core muscle training, especially for anyone who has weak or underused abdominals.

I don't believe in weight training for running. Building muscles that you don't use while running will only increase your muscle mass, creating more weight you'll have to carry around. No thanks, I'll pass on that. I practice T'ai Chi for cross-training my core muscles and focusing my mind. Spend your time on weights if you need strength for something else or if one of your goals in life is to be a chick magnet. If your doctor tells you it's necessary to build stronger muscles so you can recover from an injury, that's fine. But be sure you're *also* working on improving your running form, since it's what probably caused the injury to begin with. It is also important for older runners (50+) to do some weight training to maintain muscle mass. If you're recovering from an injury I have suggested exercises in Chapter 9, "Troubleshooting: Injury Prevention and Recovery."

If your ligaments and tendons aren't as flexible as they should be, or if certain muscles needed in your running are weak, enhance your workouts with specific cross-training until your body can get up to speed. Just know that a great way to get your whole body to work well is to strengthen and stretch it *while you're running*.

Program Upgrades: When, How, How Much

For anything to evolve to its next appropriate level of existence, for it to grow, it needs to be prodded or stretched out of its state of equilibrium into a state of imbalance, at which time the forces of Nature are engaged to create a new state of equilibrium at a new level.

If this premise is true, then balance and growth cannot exist simultaneously, because balance implies a state of equilibrium, or non-movement, and growth implies a state of movement. This may all sound very heady and esoteric, but it applies directly to your running. Here's how.

Let's say you've been religiously doing all of your ChiRunning focuses and you've gotten to the point where you can run at a nice relaxed pace, whistling pop tunes. Your body has been so used to running at this pace for so long that your runs feel pretty relaxed and effortless. In essence, you've reached a nice state of equilibrium. You might feel at home and balanced in this state. So you say to yourself, "This is okay, but I'd like to get a little faster." What do you do?

As explained in Chapter 4, if you want to go faster, all you have to do is *lean* more. So then you go out for your next run and try to lean more. What happens? If you're doing it right, you'll feel like you're tipping more forward than you're used to. You're off balance a bit and it'll probably feel somewhat uncomfortable. But with each progressive run it gets easier because Nature is doing its part by providing you with stronger abdominal muscles to handle this new angle of lean. After some weeks or maybe months, you find yourself running along with a new lean, still whistling pop tunes, just like you used to except now you're running faster. In essence, your running evolves because you introduce a state of imbalance where one hadn't existed before. Your body makes the necessary adjustments, and presto, you end up in a new state of balance that is a step above your original state—you've grown.

That's what growth is all about. It doesn't come when things are status quo. It happens only when something new is introduced, forcing every integral part to adjust. This is a universal law that can be applied on any level of life, whether it's expanding a business or helping a shy person become a better public speaker.

I don't want to imply that you're growing just because you're in a state of imbalance, but the possibility of growth is there. Too many people live most of their lives in an unbalanced state and never get anywhere.

To get this law to work for you, you must come from a balanced state and make a conscious choice to improve it. *You* choose when to stretch yourself and create the necessary state of imbalance (think Tiger Woods). Your job is to make the adjustments required to move you forward (such as really working on holding that lean). Once you choose to grow, you'll be amazed at how the forces of Nature line up to help you complete the job. Balance and growth are two of the main principles that keep Nature ticking along in that wonderful way.

THE PHILOSOPHY OF UPGRADES:
AN ADVANCED LESSON IN
THE PRINCIPLE OF BALANCE

One of the most important ways to build your running program safely is to know when and how much to upgrade. As your conditioning increases, your breath rate will relax and your core muscles won't be as tired. Maintaining a consistent lean won't be as difficult. Your shoulders and hips will feel looser and your footsteps lighter. As all of these improvements take place, your running will feel easier, and at some point you will have a choice to make. You can either plateau for a period of time, or you can upgrade your program.

A *plateau* is an important and natural part of any growth process. It is the period of time necessary for your physical development to catch up with the changes taking place in your running form. Your body needs time to get used to the fact that some muscles are being used more and some less. It's an adjustment on the cellular level, and it takes time. My 9-year-old daughter goes through growth spurts in which she'll gain an inch in a month, and then there'll be no change for a couple of weeks while the rest of her body catches up with her bone growth.

An *upgrade* is any increase in your current running program beyond what you are currently doing. Upgrading your program is a bigger deal than you might think. Any quantitative increase in your speed, distance, technique, or number of runs will increase duress to your body—namely, your muscles, ligaments, tendons, bones, heart, and lungs. For this reason it is crucial that you hold your upgrades to no more than two per week.

GENERAL GUIDELINES FOR UPGRADING A RUNNING PROGRAM

- Don't make more than two upgrades of any kind per week.
- Don't add more than fifteen to thirty seconds on to an interval.
- Don't add more than fifteen minutes (or 10% additional mileage) to a long run each week.
- If you increase the number of intervals, run the earlier ones slightly slower.
- If you increase the speed at which you run your intervals, decrease the total number, then slowly build the number weekly while maintaining your new speed.
- If you happen to have a good run when you unexpectedly run faster or farther than usual, don't follow it with any scheduled upgrades. Postpone them until the following week.

Upgrades that are not well thought out and prepared for are the number one cause of running injuries. This is called overtraining, the general term used to describe running at a level beyond what your body is capable of. It occurs in all classes of runners, from beginners to elites. If you try to run 2 miles on your very first run, you could be easily injured in a number of ways. If there are weaknesses in your running form, the potential for injury magnifies as the miles increase. Build slowly and let your body knowledge grow gradually until you can add upgrades without defaulting back into how you used to run. If you're a beginning runner, your first upgrades will be adding more minutes to your runs. The next upgrade will be form intervals.

As you get a clearer understanding and body experience of the ChiRunning focuses, you will be able to sense within yourself what you most need to upgrade and when to do it. Go by feel.

Here is a list of possible upgrades.

- Increase the speed of a specific run.
- Increase the number of interval repeats. (Increase your interval workout by no more than one interval per week, and add one only if your body says it's okay.)
- Increase the length of each interval.
- Increase the overall time of a run.
- Increase the steepness or length of a hill run.
- Increase the number of your weekly runs. (This is a big step and not to be taken lightly. Any additional weekly run should always be a fun run at first. Allow yourself a couple of weeks to transition into the additional day per week before introducing any specific theme into the run.)

HOW TO TELL WHEN YOU NEED AN UPGRADE

Body Sensing, Body Sensing, Body Sensing. You guessed it—you can do it when your body says it's okay. If you try to push an upgrade before your body is ready, you're asking for trouble. Any upgrades need to be proposed by your mind but ratified by your body, kind of like the House and Senate.

The best time to check in with your body is toward the end of the run that you plan to upgrade. As you approach the close of your scheduled workout, ask yourself, "Could I do another ___ right now?" (Fill in the blank with the appropriate increment: 1 interval, 1 mile, 15 minutes, 30 seconds, whatever.) If you listen carefully to your body, it will give you one of three responses when you ask it to do more:

A) "Sure, no problem."

B) "Yeah, I **could** do it. I'm a little tired, but I think I've got it in me."

C) "No way, I'm outta here!"

If your body answers with A or B, you have the green light for an upgrade. Anything in the C range is out of the question. Give it another week before asking again.

Even if you have scheduled an upgrade for a given week, you should upgrade only if it's appropriate to your conditioning.

The beauty of this method is that it has the built-in safety mechanism of Body Sensing, which, if used properly, will never allow you to be injured due to a premature upgrade. Warning: Body Sensing is easily cut off by the ego (your mind). Keep a good back-and-forth dialogue happening with your body, and it will always let you know what's okay and what's not.

If you follow this approach, you may be amazed at what your body can do over time. Here's a testimonial from a client who's been practicing the ChiRunning technique for seven years.

From a purely physical viewpoint, ChiRunning can be used to run faster and farther and will definitely make one a better and more relaxed runner. However, I feel that there is so much more to it than that. By practicing the principles of Body Sensing and efficiently using my muscle energy to enjoy my runs, it teaches me that I can learn to sense myself physically and emotionally in all situations and to not waste energy as I journey through life. Incorporating this philosophy with a holistic focus enables me to achieve a true sense of peace and happiness.

Aga Goodsell

ILLNESS AND RUNNING

I don't run when I have a fever, when I'm in the contagious stage of a cold, or when I'm sick and the temperature is below freezing. But otherwise, I'm out there, because it gets my heart pumping, my lungs expanding, and my lymphatic system circulating, not to mention my chi flowing. Again, if you can Body Sense what you need, you'll do fine. If you are recovering from or dealing with a more serious illness, you need to Body Sense, check in with your health practitioner and lean toward building and preserving your health. Running may help you manage or improve some health conditions, but you do not want to deplete yourself while healing.

SHOES AND EQUIPMENT

SHOES

One of the things I love about running is its simplicity. For the most part it's just a matter of putting on your running clothes and heading out the door. As you start training for longer distances and racing, it's a good idea to put some thoughtful attention into your clothing and equipment. In terms of equipment, the only things we highly recommend are good shoes, a metronome, a watch with a countdown timer, and a running log. Running is one of the best ways to get healthy and fit and also keep it simple.

Intelligent Feet

I once went into Chinatown in San Francisco to buy a pair of T'ai Chi shoes. When I told the Chinese woman behind the counter what I wanted, she took one look at the running shoes I had on and said, "I don't understand why you Westerners wear shoes like *that* . . . all they do is make your feet stupid."

I was so taken by surprise with her candidness and accuracy that my only response was, "Guilty as charged." She was talking about the fact that most running shoes are so overbuilt and have such thick soles that they prevent us from feeling the ground beneath us. When practicing T'ai Chi it is crucial to maintain a very direct contact with the ground in order to feel "rooted" and stable. So it is mandatory to have very flexible, thin-soled shoes.

An important aspect to keep in mind when practicing Chi-Running or ChiWalking is that you're trying to build intelligent movement into your body—which to a surprisingly large degree is informed by the intelligence in your feet. As your feet train your body how to have the best postural alignment, you'll enjoy good flexibility and mobility, and maintain healthy feet, legs, and posture for a lifetime.

Your Shoes Can Hurt You

For years now, as a response to the high injury rate of runners, shoe manufacturers have been designing shoes with increasingly thicker heels. But even though they have tried their best to solve the problem by designing better shoes, the annual rate of running injuries has not dropped. There are now studies showing that the thicker heels are creating an earlier and more sustained contact with the ground, increasing impact to the legs, knees, and joints. If you want to find a pair of shoes without an elevated heel, ask for "training flats," which are generally designed for runners who have better biomechanics than most runners. Some shoe manufacturers are now designing a midfoot strike shoe, so ask your local running shoe store if they carry any.

If you have problems with your feet, read about exercises to help in Chapter 9, "Troubleshooting: Injury Prevention and Recovery."

Barefoot Running

There has been a remarkable amount of press about running barefoot. I personally prefer finding a great shoe, but the reason why I support the concept is that running barefoot is the single fastest way to find out how good your form really is. Barefoot runners don't heel-strike, because the foot is "educating" the body about how you should make contact with the ground. For most of us, this can be a harsh reality if we take away our shoes.

People who run barefoot as a rule have much better running form than people who wear shoes. Go to your local track sometime and run a lap without your shoes on, and see what happens to your running form. You'll come back a non-heel-striker. Running barefoot forces you to land on that nice, soft midsection of your foot instead of your heel. It also forces you to lean forward, keeping your weight in front of where your feet strike the ground. This is an example of your feet teaching your body how to run correctly. Try it and you'll be convinced. Less is better.

Rather than running barefoot, I run almost entirely in racing flats. They have the least built-up heel, the least amount of structure and cushioning, and the greatest amount of flexibility. You too will be running in racing flats when you learn to always have a soft, midfoot landing, with no heel strike or toe-off, and you can clearly Body Sense the difference.

Buying Shoes

Here's a brief guide to buying a great pair of running shoes.

Comfort: First and foremost, choose a shoe that is comfortable. It should fit like a glove in the heel section, with no sense of cramping in the toe box. Go to your local friendly running store and ask the salesperson to bring you shoes in your size that are flexible and lightweight. No clunkers here. Try them all on to see how they fit. You're looking for a shoe that has plenty of room for your toes. They should never be touching the front of the toe box, and your feet should not feel squeezed at all. The more they feel like bedroom slippers, the better.

Flexibility: The next thing you're looking for is flexibility. Hold the shoe with one hand on the front and the other hand on the heel, and bend it in the same motion it would bend as you run (figure 63). Watch carefully for where it bends. If it's a good shoe, it will bend right at the ball area (just aft of the toebox). If it bends in the middle, it will overstretch the muscles on the bottom of your foot (and cause plantar fasciitis). If it doesn't bend and feels rather stiff over the length of the sole, forget it. A shoe that doesn't flex well will throw you onto your toes, causing your calves to overwork as you roll forward off your foot at the end of your stride. No thank you.

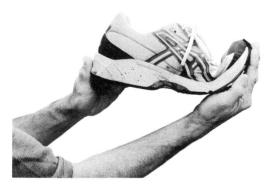

Figure 63—Flexing the shoe

Light weight: Look for a shoe that has some cushioning but is lightweight. Some shoe stores keep a scale on hand. If the shoes weigh in over 14 ounces for a medium-size foot, forget it; you're not looking for combat boots. A good training flat should weigh in under 11 ounces and preferably 8 to 9. Generally speaking, the more a shoe weighs, the stiffer it is, so ask for racing flats or training flats. If you've just started your ChiRunning program and are used to lots of support from your shoes, you can slowly transition into softer and lighter shoes as your form improves. A more neutral shoe trains your *foot* to do what is necessary for your running, instead of relying on the shoe to do all the work.

Stock up: If you find a pair of shoes that really works well for you, *you* can rest assured they won't be around in six months. So go for it and buy three or four pairs if your budget can handle it. Finding a good shoe is like finding an honest mechanic—when it happens, it's like striking gold.

Trail Shoes: If you're a trail runner, you'll need a shoe with an aggressive sole, meaning that it has lugs to improve traction on dirt surfaces. But be careful; shoes that are labeled "trail shoes" are generally pretty stiff and overbuilt. Look for a pair that allows your foot to ride somewhat low to the ground and has a slightly snugger fit so your foot isn't slipping around in the shoe with all the lateral motion of trail running.

Because shoe styles change so frequently, we can't suggest specific shoes here, but we do have regular updates on running shoes at our website.

Breaking In a Pair of Running Shoes

When you buy a new pair of running shoes, take some time to break them in; don't just throw them on and take off on your long run. Let your body adjust to the new shoes, and let the shoes adjust to you. Follow the principle of Gradual Progress and take it slowly. Don't do more than about 3 miles on your first outing. After that, the general rule that I follow is not to run over twice the distance of my last run on the new pair. For instance, if your last run on the new shoes was 3 miles, you shouldn't go over 6 miles on the next run.

How to Tell When You Need New Shoes

When you take a new pair of running shoes out of the box, write the date on the rear of the shoe with a permanent marker. After you've been running on that pair of shoes for four months, be on the lookout for any stress in your legs (above and beyond the normal) during or after your runs. If the pavement feels a little bit harder or the trails are wearing your legs out more than usual, switch to a new pair of shoes. If those sensations go away with the first run in the new shoes, you've made a good choice. If nothing changes, go back and read Chapter 4. If you log your miles, you should switch shoes after about 500 miles. That number will increase as your running gets smoother and more fluid. I have gotten as much as 750 miles on a pair of racing flats, but that's more the exception than the rule.

Also periodically check the soles of your shoes for excessive wear spots and replace any shoes that are worn through to the midsole.

Keeping Your Shoes Tied

How many times have you double-knotted your laces to keep them from coming untied only to be unable to adjust them in the midst of a run because of cold fingers? If you're tired of your shoes coming untied, here are two ways to eliminate the problem forever. (1) After making the first loop with your laces, wrap the other lace around the loop *twice* instead of once, then finish tying the bow. If you want to untie your shoes, simply pull on the lace ends, and ta-da! (2) Tie your shoes in a regular bow and then take both loops, hold them together, and tuck them under one of the laces farther down on the shoe. My shoes have *never* come untied with this one, and it also keeps my loops from getting caught on branches, which is a real drag (so to speak). This method also allows you to untie the laces with a simple pull.

SPORTS WATCH

This is an essential tool to improve your running. Along with the metronome, which is a key tool in ChiRunning and ChiWalking, the other important accessory is a good watch. We recommend a digital watch with a chronometer, a single and double countdown timer, and

30–50-lap memory. We sell one on our website that is the best watch we've found for our purposes.

As you get to know what your watch can do, you'll find that you'll be able to create workouts that are fun and interesting to do.

- **Fifty-lap memory** lets you note the duration and date of up to fifty runs or up to fifty splits. If you don't get to your running log right after a run, this feature can keep track of the days and length of your runs; it can also keep track of splits in a race or a run. In ChiRunning we recommend that you start slowly and gradually increase your speed as your body warms up and relaxes more. The lap memory is a great way to see if your speed increases as you relax.
- **The repeat countdown timer** is a great tool for simple intervals. You can set the beeper to go off every two minutes as a reminder to check in with a Form Focus you are practicing. As we all know, it is easy to get distracted and let our mind wander. The countdown timer is a gentle reminder to return your mind to the Form Focus.
- **The dual countdown timer** lets you get more sophisticated with your Form Focus practices and is an essential tool for intervals. You can set the first timer for two to three minutes and the second one for one minute. Then work on your Form Focus for two to three minutes followed by one minute off to just relax.

  This also works for building cardiovascular strength. Go faster for two to three minutes, getting your heart rate up, then take a one-minute recovery break at a slower pace to let your heart rate slow down. Then increase again for two to three minutes, and so on.
- **Check your heart rate** with the basic chronometer. Holding two fingers against your neck just under your lower jaw, check your pulse rate over a one-minute period. This is a low-tech way to check your heart rate. As a baseline reference point, it is important to know your resting heart rate (RHR)—see Chapter 6, page 146. As your level of conditioning improves, you will notice a drop in this number, so it's good to check occasionally so that you can chart your progress toward better health.
- **The hourly beeper** is a reminder throughout the day to stop

and check in, with posture, with Body Sensing, with ourselves. If you know you slouch at your desk, it can be a reminder to sit up straight. Use it to drink water, take a two-minute computer break—whatever is going to help you most.

Metronome

In Chapter 4, I talked about how to use the metronome to learn gears and cadence. This is the single best piece of equipment I can recommend to help your running form. Creating a rhythmic stride is by far the best way to learn the ChiRunning form and it's easy to do because your body loves rhythms. The metronome is the best tool for learning how to lengthen or shorten your stride relative to your speed.

Heart Rate Monitor

If you have health issues or are tracking your heart rate for specific reasons, then by all means use a heart rate monitor. But for most people, I don't think a heart rate monitor is necessary. I prefer that you learn to Body Sense what your perceived rate of exertion is, rather than depend on a monitor to tell you. Learn to sense what an appropriate level of a workout feels like.

I do have one great use for a heart rate monitor: as a biofeedback tool. The concept is to see if you can decrease your heart rate while running a steady pace or to see if you can run slightly faster without increasing your heart rate. The idea is to find efficiency through working on your running form. Here's what you do: Warm up for at least fifteen minutes. When you have leveled off at a steady pace, start your heart rate monitor. Then either (1) hold that pace and try to reduce your heart rate by working on some aspect of your form (such as lean, relaxation, or rotating your hips), or (2) try to increase your pace while maintaining the same heart rate by working on your form.

GPS Systems

I don't have one of those GPS systems for runners. If you want to know every detail about your run—how far, how fast, exactly where you've been—then by all means, indulge yourself. If you're training for a marathon, I think it would be very handy for keeping track of your various course distances and your pace. I borrowed one once and had fun making a map of the trails I ran. You can use the GPS to monitor your pace, which is helpful when you're learning pacing. Just be aware that the pace it shows will be only an approximation and not as accurate as timing yourself at track or on a measured course.

That being said, I think they can be a distraction if you overfocus on results. I think it's important to get a feel for things inside your own body rather than relying on equipment all the time. I have gotten to know my own pacing so well, I know it within seconds per mile. If you do have a GPS system, my main suggestion would be to listen to your body first, then consult with your GPS. Use it as a tool to get to know your running better from the inside out, rather than the outside in.

Water Belts and Hydration Packs

Today, there are many types of belts and hydration systems; you'll need to shop around to find out which works best for you. As an ultra runner, I do have quite a collection. My favorite one holds a 20-ounce water bottle at an angle at my lower back. I like it because it's easy to slip the water bottle in and out.

What is important here is to stay adequately hydrated, especially for long-distance running or races, so get used to running with either a belt or a hydration pack. Even if you're training for a marathon with a group that provides water stops, I still recommend that you train with a water belt. I'll talk more about this and hydration in Chapter 10, "Peak Performance and Race-Specific Training."

CHAPTER SEVEN

Hills, Trails, and Treadmills

It does not matter how slowly you go so long as you do not stop. —CONFUCIUS

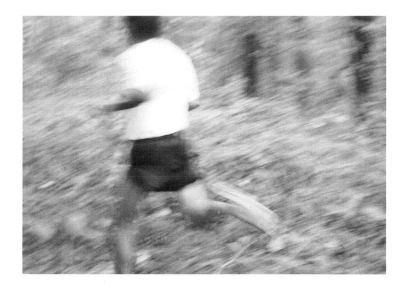

One of the best aspects of running is that the environmental conditions in which you run are constantly changing. Like a T'ai Chi Master, you can learn to respond to every situation in the best way possible. As you become thoroughly familiar and comfortable with the basics of the ChiRunning technique you will begin to respond intuitively without having to think at all. Hills, trails, and treadmills are great opportunities to expand your basic ChiRunning skills and use them in a wider variety of circumstances.

HILLS—FLOAT AND FLOW

Running hills (especially trails) is my all-time favorite type of running. There's something very satisfying about cresting a hill and looking back on what I've climbed. Running uphill gives me a great cardiovascular workout without having to add any speed, and running downhill allows me to practice my smoothness and flow. It's so exhilarating to fly down a mountain trail, passing rocks and trees like they're standing still.

Many people shy away from hills, thinking they're too much work. But let me clue you in on a little secret—they're not that much more work if you can learn to run them with *technique* instead of muscles. Just think of hills as another opportunity to practice your gears, and you'll find yourself using a lot less effort on your way up. And, you can use downhill running as a great way to learn to relax and go with the flow. With the ChiRunning technique you use your upper body more on the uphills and your lower body more on the downhills. I'll explain this more as we go.

Running hills is very different from running on level ground. So if you're just beginning to learn ChiRunning, the best advice I can give you is to practice your new running technique on flat ground before attempting to run hills. If you start running hills while you're still learning the basics of technique, you could easily default into "muscling" your way up those hills and then pounding your legs on the downhills.

> **Injury Prevention Tip.** Whenever you set out to run hills of any kind, always take the time to warm up on *flat* terrain before heading up any incline. This allows you to implement your basic running focuses and have them integrated into your movement *before* any terrain challenges come up. It also allows your muscles time to warm up and get blood flowing, reducing your odds of overstretching a tendon.

As the old saying goes, "There are exceptions to every rule." This holds true for the basic rules of ChiRunning. All the ChiRunning focuses are meant as general guidelines for efficient running on a level surface. Some of the "rules" change when you start running hills. In this section we'll cover all the hill running focuses. I'll point out which rules you get to break, and at the end of this section I'll list them all for you.

Uphill Running

ChiRunning not only makes running on the flats easier, it also makes running up hills easier. When you're running on a flat surface, think of your body as a team of two—upper body and lower body—with a 50/50 shared responsibility of moving you along the road. When running uphill with the ChiRunning technique you'll need to increase the emphasis on your upper body (more like 60/40 or 70/30) to take some of the workload off your legs. It's not just a matter of increasing your upper body effort; it actually means *reducing* your lower body effort. Whenever I come to an uphill stretch, I always think of getting a great upper body workout but *resting* my legs!

For this reason, there are two things you exaggerate on the uphills: your lean and your arm swing. In the next two sections I'll explain the differences between running up moderate hills and steep hills.

RUNNING UP EASY TO MODERATE HILLS

- **Lean into the hill.** Lean forward into the hill, keeping your shoulders slightly ahead of your hips as you run. Here's why. When you are running on a level surface, you're leaning forward. As a hill comes up in front of you, it may throw you back into an upright position, which will cause you to step up the hill in front of your body. This overworks your hamstrings because you're reaching up the hill with every step and *pulling* yourself up the hill. To counteract this tendency, lean into the hill and keep your upper body ahead of your hips and feet. You will feel like you're leaning more because you'll sense an increased tension in your Achilles tendons. That's because the hill is coming up in front of you.
- **Don't step ahead of your hips.** In order to prevent the overuse of your hamstrings, never step past your hips when running uphill. As you lean into the hill keep your shoulders *ahead* of your hips and your hips *ahead* of your feet.

- **Swing your arms *forward and up*.** Since you won't be using your legs as much, your upper body will have to pick up the slack. When running uphill, your arms should swing *forward*, not to the rear as in flat running. (This is where you get to break the rule about always swinging your arms to the rear.) Bring your hands closer in to your body and swing them in an upward motion, from your hips to your chin. Pretend you're trying to punch yourself in the chin. It should feel like you're doing an uppercut, like a boxer. This is a great way to get an upper body workout, which most runners hardly ever get.

- **Shorten your stride length.** The best way to reduce your lower body effort on hills is to relax everything below your waist as much as possible. This naturally shortens your stride length and shifts you into a lower gear. Isn't that what you do in your car when you go uphill? In order to run uphill efficiently, your body has to follow the same laws of physics that any machine would. So downshift and head up those hills using your "lower gears." If you feel fatigue in your legs, shorten your stride until you feel less fatigue. Running up hills is not the time to be in a hurry, so take it easy and you'll get to the top in great shape, without feeling like you're dying a slow death.

- **Relax your lower legs.** Keep your lower legs as relaxed as possible when running uphill. This will ensure that you don't run uphill on your toes and overwork your calf and foot muscles.

- **Keep your heels down.** In order to avoid overworking your lower leg muscles, always keep your heels on the ground during the support phase of your stride. Any time spent on your forefoot is energy spent working your *small* leg muscles to do a *big* job.

- **Use a mental image.** A good mental image to use when running uphill is to imagine yourself floating up the hills like you're a hot air balloon, or let your upper body feel spacious and light, like an eagle catching an updraft. As a friend once told me, "Why should I work to get somewhere I could float to?" Just think to yourself, "Uphill . . . upper body."

Exercise: Practice Your Efficiency on Hills

Whenever you're running up easy to moderate hills, always have the intention to try to get up the hill *without increasing your breath rate.* You might not be able to do it right away, but having this intention guide your movements will force you to focus on doing everything in your power to *not* increase your energy expenditure. Hill-running efficiency is all in your gears, lean, and upper body usage.

You can also use your heart rate monitor, if you have one, as a great biofeedback tool. Work with all the uphill focuses and try to keep your heart rate from significantly increasing as you go up.

Doing all of the above focuses will reduce your perceived rate of exertion and leave you feeling that running up hills isn't any more difficult than running on a flat surface. Your mission whenever you're running up a hill is to get to the top with as little leg usage as possible! This image will ensure that you engage your upper body and your lean so you don't overwork your legs.

RUNNING UP STEEP HILLS

If you like running hills, you'll eventually come upon one that seems like a "walker." The reason steep hills are so tiring is that keeping your heels down is difficult. Many people run up steep hills on their toes to prevent their Achilles tendons from overstretching. This overworks your shins and calves because you're using the *smaller* muscles of your legs to do a larger portion of the work, not the most efficient way to get yourself up a hill.

There's a way around this scenario: run sideways. That's right, turn your body slightly to one side and run up the hill sideways. (This is where you get to break the rule about facing your body in the direction you're headed.) When your feet turn sideways to the hill, the tension in your Achilles will go away, your heels will stay down, and your calves and shins can relax. Your feet will be doing a tiny crossover step. I call it the Lateral Stride. The beauty of this unconventional technique is that it engages your medial and lateral muscles. These muscles are generally not used much when you're on level ground, so it's like having a fresh set of muscles available to help you out. Using

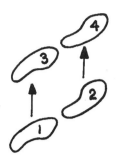

Figure 65—The "dance chart" for the Lateral Stride

these muscles also gives your quads and hamstrings a break on the uphills.

How do you tell when to do the Lateral Stride? Body Sense it. As soon as you start to feel any tension in your Achilles tendons and your heels want to come up off the ground during the support phase of your stride, turn your body (and feet) to the side just enough to eliminate the tension in your Achilles tendons and allow your heels to remain on the ground. The steeper the hill, the more sideways your feet (and body) will need to turn.

Here is the technique for running up steep hills:

• **Run sideways.** As you start up a steep hill, turn your body facing toward ten o'clock for six to eight strides, then switch to the opposite side, facing two o'clock for six to eight more strides. Work your way up the hill switching back and forth in this way. This allows your medial and lateral leg muscles to alternate between working and resting as you switch directions. This technique is great for keeping your heels down when you're heading up steep, narrow trails and don't have the luxury of zigzagging.

• **Swing your downhill arm across your body.** Your arm swing will also be different on steep uphills. As you turn your body to one side, your uphill arm will swing side-

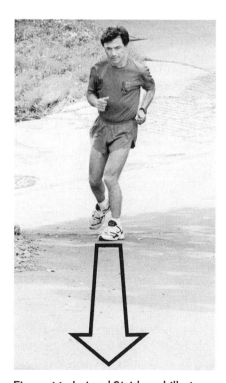

Figure 66—Lateral Stride uphill, step 1

ways relative to the slope of the hill, rendering it pretty useless. Don't worry about it. Just let it swing lightly. On the other hand (no pun intended), your downhill arm is aiming in the uphill direction, so let it swing fully across your body, reaching up for your opposite shoulder. (Here's where you get to break the rule of not crossing your centerline with your hands.)

- **Shift to "granny" gear.** Remember, it's a steep hill, so shift to your smallest gear. On the really steep hills your stride should be *shorter* than your normal first gear stride length. Slow your cadence down if you need to. (Another broken rule of keeping the same cadence.) Don't be in a hurry. Take your time heading up the steep ones.
- **Lean into the hill with your uphill shoulder.** Since your body is turned to one side or the other, you'll be leaning into the hill with your uphill shoulder. Lean with enough intent to feel as if you're leaning your shoulder into a door to break it open.

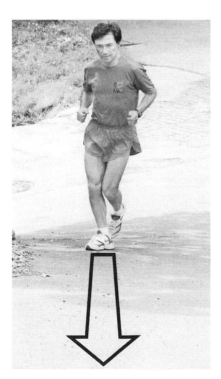 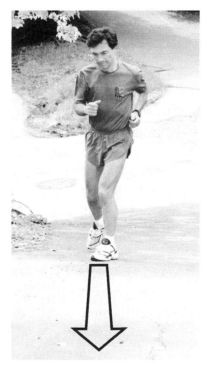

Figure 67—Lateral Stride uphill, step 2

Figure 68—Lateral Stride uphill, step 3

- **Walk if you need to.** Don't forget, if a hill is too steep to sustain any sort of running, you *always* have the option of walking. I do it all the time.

I've received my fair share of weird looks from runners when I mention going uphill sideways, until they try it. Then those looks turn to sighs of relief when they see how easy it is to run this way up a steep hill. I've even had clients say that it was the single most important thing they learned, because they no longer fear hills of any grade. That alone is worth it.

DOWNHILL RUNNING

When you're running downhill your running form will be a lot different than on the way up. As soon as you shift from running flat or uphill into running downhill, you need to switch the emphasis to your *lower body*. Your legs and pelvis are your shock absorbers, so it is their job to minimize the force of the road coming up at you. It is especially important that you neutralize the impact on the downhill, because you'll be hitting the ground with more force than on level ground (six to ten times your body weight).

The key to comfortable, smooth downhill running is knowing how to relax, both physically and mentally. Having tense muscles on the downhill increases the impact to your knees and quads, and it'll wear you out more quickly. Learning how to mentally relax while running downhill is really the more difficult aspect, because for many people it's when they run their fastest speeds.

When you take the fear out of downhill running, you'll see that it's really one of the most enjoyable aspects of running. My mind can't think as fast as my body, so I have to just let go, relax, and trust that my feet will land in the best spot . . . and they usually always do. It feels like stream-of-consciousness running, where my body takes over and my mind shuts off.

THE TWO TYPES OF DOWNHILLS

The downhill focuses all work to lower the impact to your legs and back so you can arrive at the bottom of a hill in much the same condition as when you left the top. I split downhill running into two general categories—*runnable* and *non-runnable* downhills. Some hills are so gradual that you don't have to put on the brakes to control your speed. Those are the ones I call *runnable*. It's a time to loosen your hips, stretch out your stride, and let gravity pull you. Easy downhills are the best time to learn how to soften your body, relax, and take it easy while running at speeds you normally only dream of. Then there are the steeper downhills, where you spend most of your time slowing yourself down so things don't get out of control. These I call *non-runnable* downhills.

Runnable Downhills

Here is a list of focuses that will help you experience new levels of speed and looseness on those easy downhills.

- **Relax everything from the waist down.** Pay special attention to relaxing your quads and calves.
- **Keep your cadence steady.** Let your stride length increase.
- **Lean downhill.** On the easy slopes, keep your upper body ahead of your foot strike. Holding the "C" shape is the best way to accomplish this. Regulate your speed with your lean. If you get going too fast, just let off the gas pedal and go easier. The importance of the "C" shape is that too many runners pull their shoulders back when running downhill. This puts more curvature into your lower back, increases the pressure on your sacrum and lumbar spine, and throws your legs too far forward, which makes you land hard on your heels. If you hold your body in the "C" shape with a level pelvis, it will flatten your lower back and reduce the impact to your sacrum.
- **Let your pelvis rotate more.** Let your entire lower body swing from T12/L1, allowing your pelvis to rotate with each stride. Every time your leg swings out the back, let your hip be pulled back with it. This allows your stride to open up behind you reducing the shock to your knees and quads.

- **Relax your ankles.** To avoid shin splints or plantar fasciitis from running downhill, it is crucial that you don't dorsiflex your ankles (see photo on page 107). I sometimes point my toes as my legs swing forward to avoid a hard heel strike.
- **Relax your mind.** Surrender to the speed, Grasshopper.

Non-runnable Downhills

Whenever you find yourself "putting on the brakes" on a downhill, it's your body telling you that a change in technique is in order. Here is a list of focuses that will transform those steep downhills into something fun and relaxing.

- **Control your speed with your "gas pedal."** When your car goes down a steep hill, let off on the gas pedal, right? If your lean is your gas pedal, then let it return to vertical on the steep downhills.
- **Take very small strides** and peel up your heels with each step, instead of coming down onto your feet with your whole weight. This focus alone will significantly reduce the amount of impact to your quads and feet. If you want to run down a steep hill faster, simply pick up your heels faster; your cadence will increase but you won't increase the impact to your legs.
- **Zigzag** down the hill if there's enough room. This will allow your lateral muscles to do some of the work of shock absorption.
- **Relax your shoulders** and keep them low. If you need stability, hold your hands out away from your

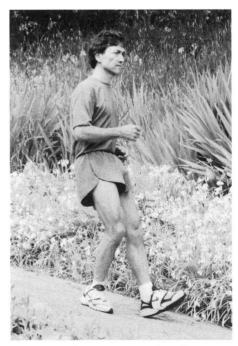

Figure 69—Posture vertical, tailbone tucked, soft heel strike

sides. In addition to relaxing your shoulders remember to relax your whole body, especially your legs, and the ride down will be much softer.

• **Balance yourself** in a vertical position directly over your ankles and let your weight ride softly on your heels (figure 69). This will direct the shock absorption to the back side of your legs. As your foot comes down, roll heel-to-toe to further reduce impact.

If you're familiar with the ChiWalking technique, going down very steep hills is the only time when all the focuses of ChiRunning and ChiWalking are an identical match.

Exercise: Leg Strengthening for Downhills

Here's a T'ai Chi stance that will strengthen your legs for the down-hills. Begin with a Grounding Stance (figure 70). Then stand with one leg in front of the other (figure 71). All of your weight should be on the leg that is under your body. Bend your knee slightly, keeping a

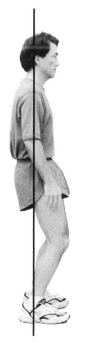

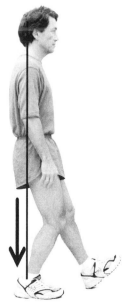

Figure 71—Shift weight to one leg, drop tailbone to heel

Figure 70—Grounding stance

straight, vertical line between your ear, shoulder, hip, and ankle. Keep your forward leg relaxed with your heel resting on the ground but not supporting your weight. Stand this way every day for one to two minutes if you can, then change legs and do it for one to two minutes on the other leg. Pretend you have an invisible support leg running from your heel to your tailbone. As your legs become stronger, you'll be able to handle more time on each one. This is the single most effective exercise that has helped me to improve my downhill running speed and reduced the impact to my quads.

Here's a list of all the ChiRunning rules you get to break when you run hills:

Gradual Uphills
- More upper body work, less lower body work
- Hold hands close to your chest—at less than a 90° angle
- Swing arms forward and up instead of rearward

Steep Uphills
- Lean with your uphill shoulder
- Downhill arm crosses your centerline
- Body faces to the side, not forward
- Decrease your cadence if you need to

Runnable Downhill
- Point your toes as your legs swing forward (this prevents dorsiflexion)

Non-runnable Downhills
- No lean . . . posture vertical
- Pick up your knees (slightly)
- Land on the front of your heels and roll heel-to-toe
- Stride length shortens
- Cadence *increases* as your speed increases

As a general rule when running hills, feel the chi in your body rising when you go uphill, and feel it descending when you're running downhill. Whenever you find yourself surrounded by hills, just think, "Float and flow." You'll find that it's a very body-friendly way to take to the hills.

TRAIL RUNNING: A HEALTHY ADDICTION

Of all the types of running I do, I'd have to say that my hands-down favorite is trail running. It's a time when I can truly become thoughtless, in the best sense of the term. My mind can be at peace while my body gets relaxed and energized. I spent over half my life running in the mountains above Boulder, Colorado. Then I lived in Marin County, California, and ran the Marin Headlands for ten years. Now I live in the Blue Ridge Mountains and enjoy the trails every day. I feel blessed to have lived in three of the most ideal places for trail running.

The reason why trail running is such a fabulous experience for me is because running in natural surroundings takes me beyond the running itself. Running on mountain trails is where my spirit thrives and I'm in touch with Nature through the four seasons. Passing through a living, constantly changing environment builds my technical skills and awakens all of my senses. My mind quiets and my body and instincts take over, like an animal running through the woods.

As a kid, didn't you love to play make-believe, that you were an explorer or an Indian runner with a message for the chief? Trail running still does that for me. It is pure play and pure freedom.

One of my favorite running scenes ever caught on film is at the beginning of the movie *The Last of the Mohicans*. I love watching the sheer agility and abandonment of an Indian flying through a forest in pursuit of a deer. It's also one of Katherine's favorite scenes because it's Daniel Day-Lewis doing the running.

THE PHYSICAL BENEFITS OF TRAIL RUNNING

Trails, by their nature, follow the lay of the land, which is why I consider them the most challenging type of running. They challenge you to shift your focus and adapt in a split second. They require more focus and more skill, but as you'll see, not necessarily more strength.

Trails are the perfect place to practice mastering your ChiRunning technique because they require good balance, stability, and fluidity. There's no better way to strengthen what needs to be strengthened and loosen what needs to be loosened.

If you're new to running hilly trails, I suggest finding a trail with a very easy incline—the more gradual, the better. It's also worth reminding you to be sure to warm up on flat terrain before heading up. As you start up your first incline, make note of the time on your watch. If you have a stopwatch, hit the start button. Start off by running up the trail using your uphill ChiRunning focuses until your legs feel some fatigue, which is perfectly normal. Make note of how much time it took to run up to this point. Then, turn around and run back down the hill, practicing your downhill focuses back to the base of the hill. Repeat this cycle until your body tells you that you're done for the day, then cool down and end your workout. Doing hill repeats in this way will gradually introduce your body to trail running without leaving you tired and discovering that you're two miles from where you started. As you're able to run longer uphills, you'll begin to have a built-in sense of how far you can let yourself go and still have plenty of energy left to get yourself back home.

Relax Your Legs and Ankles

Many runners have a tendency to tense up their legs and ankles when they feel unstable because they want to maintain control of their balance. Doing this actually makes you *less* adaptable to the terrain and increases your amount of impact with the ground. If you stiffen your legs and ankles, you're more likely to roll an ankle, jam your knees, or pound your quads, none of which is very much fun. Running with softer knees and ankles allows your body to naturally gravitate toward its own support and alignment system while softening your ride. Check in with your body as you're running. If you find yourself holding tension anywhere in your legs, gather to your center and let any tension flow right down into the dirt with each stride you take.

Practice Transitioning Quickly

The place where I see trail runners wasting the most energy is in the transitions between uphill and downhill and visa versa. If you're running down a hill and have to switch to a sudden uphill section, you need to switch from your downhill gear to your uphill gear in an instant. If you miss this transition, your stride will be too long when you head into the uphill slope and you'll be overworking your legs, wasting valuable energy.

Be watchful of the trail ahead and be mindful of how you need to transition between downhill focuses and uphill focuses. With practice you'll always be responding to every change in slope with the appropriate focuses.

SAFETY TIPS FOR TRAIL RUNNING

Here are some safety tips that apply specifically to trail running.

- Know where you're going. Study maps or ask questions of someone who has run the trail. Know what to expect in terms of natural dangers and physical challenges, and always be cognizant of your physical limits in terms of strength and endurance.
- If you plan to be on the trail for more than an hour, bring water. Don't rely on drinking from streams or springs.
- Wear appropriate clothing. If you're in an area that is subject to extreme weather changes, take what you think you'll need.
- If you're going on a backcountry trail alone, tell someone where you're going and when you expect to return. Even better, invite a friend to share your run with you.
- Be aware that as soon as you stop running, your body begins to cool down and lose body heat. If you're running in cool or rainy weather, plan your run so you have easy access to heat and/or dry clothing when you're finished with your run.
- Lace your shoes snugly but not tight. After tying your shoes, tuck the bows into the laces across your instep. This will keep the loops from snagging on branches and tripping you. I've been there, so this is sound advice.
- If you're running on a very rocky trail, wear cycling gloves. They

have padded palms in case you do a face plant on the trail, and the fingers of the gloves are usually cut off so you still have good use of your hands.

- If you're on rough or root-covered terrain, pick your feet up higher than usual with each step. Dance through those rocks and roots!
- When running down loose dirt trails or gravelly slopes, try to land on buried rocks or on the grassy sides of the trail. The rule of thumb is: aim your feet to land on anything that *won't* move when you step on it.
- When running in thick forests, don't run with a baseball cap (or turn it around so the bill is in back) or you could miss seeing low-hanging branches. I've been there too.

I hope you'll be able to learn from whatever mistakes and positive corrections I've made. But the best way to learn to run trails is to just get out there and do it. If you're already a trail runner, I hope I've added to your bag of tricks for enjoying trails even more.

TREADMILL RUNNING

For almost all of us, there's a time when we need to run on a tread-mill: too hot, too cold, unsafe area, time crunch, convenience. If for whatever reason you need to make friends with your local treadmill, these focuses should help. Running on the treadmill is prime time to practice many aspects of your technique.

- **Posture.** Whether you're running or walking on a treadmill, it's especially important to focus on good posture with every stride. Before you even push the start button, establish your posture from the feet up. In order to maintain good biomechanical efficiency, keep returning your focus to your posture throughout your workout. If there is a mirror nearby, use it to confirm your body alignment, while Body Sensing how it feels.
- **Lean.** The console/bar at the front of the machine gets in the way of a good lean and arm swing, so stay about an arm's length back from the bar at all times. I have found it harder to lean and get my

feet landing behind my center of mass on a treadmill. Setting your treadmill to a slight incline can help with this (start with a minimum of 1; I found 1.5 to 2.0 to be the best for me). Keep your ankles relaxed and be sure to keep your heels comfortably down on your landing.

- **Midfoot Strike.** Keep your stride quick and short and lift your feet to help minimize the impact transferred to your legs by the moving belt. Exaggerate the heel lift a bit more on the treadmill because there is no forward momentum to help your feet travel in a circular path. Be aware of not letting your foot swing forward into the oncoming belt. Instead, your feet should be landing with a midfoot strike, moving in a *rearward* direction as you make contact with the treadmill.

- **Begin by setting the speed at a slow enough pace** that you can comfortably jog while instating the ChiRunning focuses.

- **Practice pelvic rotations with each stride.** Every time your leg swings out behind you, let your hip be pulled back with it. This allows your entire lower body to rotate along your vertical axis and absorb much of the shock of your foot hitting the treadmill.

- **Use a metronome** on the treadmill to set your cadence. Most people have a very slow cadence on the treadmill—as low as 70. Keep your stride short and quick. Make achieving your optimal cadence a top priority.

- **Practice running at different speeds with the same cadence.** Mary Lindahl, one of our Master ChiRunning Instructors, explains it beautifully in this letter: "My first major 'aha' experience with ChiRunning came just after I had bought my metronome and was matching my cadence to it, while running on a treadmill. I warmed up for a mile and got used to matching my stride to the beep, then I increased the speed of the treadmill by a minute per mile. I had this unusual feeling of slowing down to continue matching the metronome, yet I knew I was running faster as the speed shown on the treadmill didn't lie. I thought, 'If I can feel like I'm slowing down yet know I'm running faster, I want this technique!' I literally got off the treadmill, went upstairs to my computer and looked for the next ChiRunning workshop. I felt lucky to have had this experience on the treadmill as I might have thought I was imagining the extra speed if I was on the open road. The beauty of the treadmill is that it can take some things that are usually variables and make them constants."

- **Practice the Lateral Stride** (see "Running Up Steep Hills," page 177). Set the treadmill to an incline of 5 and run for thirty seconds straight ahead, toward twelve o'clock. Then turn your body to the *left*—toward ten o'clock—for 30 seconds. Go back to twelve o'clock for 30 seconds, then to the *right* toward two o'clock for 30 seconds, then back to twelve o'clock again. It takes only a few minutes to get used to the feeling of running with your body turned to the side. Repeat this cycle as many times as you like. One thing that you can Body Sense is how much more difficult it is to run with your body facing forward than rotated to the side. On a treadmill you can make the grade of the hill and your running speed both constants.
- **Videotape yourself.** You can get instant feedback by setting up your video camera to observe your running gait. You can also use a mirror to get good feedback—or even use your reflection in a TV screen.
- **Watch your shoulders** to see if you're keeping them square to the front (correct) or whether you're rotating them with your arm swing (incorrect).
- **Practice running barefoot.** Run barefoot for a few minutes at a time to break any habit of heel striking. This helps you become aware of how you are landing on your feet so that you can Body Sense better when you have shoes on.
- **When you get off the treadmill, picture the earth like a treadmill.** All you have to do when you're running is pick up your feet and let the earth pass by underneath you.

Things to be careful of when practicing ChiRunning on a treadmill:

- **Be careful not to let the treadmill do too much of the work for you.** This can happen with a slow cadence because your foot is in the support phase too long. I recommend lifting your heels as quickly as possible, which results in a quicker cadence. Make achieving your optimal cadence (usually 90) a top priority if you run on a treadmill.

- **Follow the principle of Gradual Progress** when adjusting to running on a treadmill, or adjusting to the streets again after a winter of treadmill running. When first running on a treadmill, you may find it harder until you get used to balancing on the moving belt. Most people who get used to doing lots of miles on treadmills find that returning to the streets creates much more impact on their legs. Asphalt and pavement are much harder surfaces than the average treadmill surface.

- **The quality of the treadmill can cause experiences to vary.** The less expensive models have more spring to them, which may be harder to balance on in the beginning, but they also provide more cushioning. The more expensive "club" models do a better job of imitating running on the road, as they require less balancing and create less vertical displacement. They also have much more stability during faster running. The longer the treadmill the better and the easier to adopt the ChiRunning lean.

- **Log some miles on the road.** Most people say treadmills are easier on the legs than pavement or asphalt. Training on the treadmill is okay for some of the time, but it is important to mix in some mileage on the roads. Your body needs to be acclimated to concrete or asphalt, especially if you're training for a distance event.

- **Avoid doing prolonged speed work** (intervals, tempo runs, etc.) **on the treadmill.** The moving belt can introduce more impact at the landing, and that impact is magnified by speed. For safety reasons, it's just not the place to run faster than a comfortable aerobic pace. So whether you're simply maintaining your aerobic base or doing marathon training, always keep it easy on the treadmill. If you want a little more of a workout, you can slightly increase the amount of incline.

CHAPTER EIGHT

Transitioning Into and Out of Running

The beginning holds the seed of all that is to follow. —I CHING

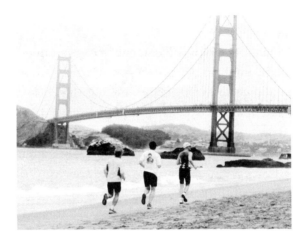

As much as I stress the importance of good running form, it's the setup and approach that dictate the *quality* of a workout. The most important part of a running program is obviously the running, but I would say that transitioning takes a very close second.

A transition is a conscious pause. It is a time to take stock of yourself and think about the run you are about to begin. The space before a run is like the pause between breaths. It's the thoughtful moment that precedes movement, when you set up your intentions of what you'd like to do during your run. It's your opportunity to ponder what you'd like to focus on, whether it's pacing, focuses, weak areas of form, recovering your legs, scouting new running routes, or just breaking in shoes.

One of my favorite times to watch elite athletes is just before a race. I imagine them playing the whole scenario of what they're about to do in their heads. They're trying to focus and relax at the same time. The ones who are most successful at doing both are the ones who are usually at the head of the pack.

Transitioning also includes the time *after* running, when you relax and review what you just did, not judging what you did, simply observing it and making note of anything that stands out. There's no such thing as a bad run, no matter how you may feel during or afterward. That's because there's always something of value that you can come away with, always a lesson to be learned if you're looking for it.

Transitioning properly into and out of your runs will not only have beneficial effects on your workouts; it can also be used as an everyday ritual that connects your running with the rest of your life, making it a sacred event, which it is.

Transitioning into a Run

PREPARING YOUR MIND

Move into every workout mentally prepared. Assess your present state and consider what you might want to do during your upcoming run. When you're getting ready to go out for a run, the following steps will make your preparation more thorough and your running practice more intentional.

- **Look at the big picture.** What type of run is on the schedule? Is there some aspect of this training run that you should pay particular attention to?
- **Body Sense or check in with yourself.** Get a clear sense of your present state. Try to feel if there is anything going on in your body that could adversely influence your run, either physically, emotionally, or mentally. Various examples could be illness, fatigue, low energy, injuries, stiff or sore muscles, a full stomach, tension or worry, time constraints—basically anything that could draw you away from having a clean, undistracted run.

- **Adjust your run** if you need to accommodate something going on in your body. For example, if you have stiff muscles, you might want to start off a bit slower and let the soreness work its way out before you pick up the speed.
- **Know specifically what you will be focusing on** so that your energy and attention are best utilized during your run. What will your focuses be? What is the most important thing for you to practice on this run? What are your intentions? What would you like to come away with?
- **Watch yourself.** Commit to checking in with your form at regular intervals. Set the countdown timer on your watch to go off every ten minutes. The beep will serve as an alarm clock bringing you back to your focuses and intentions. This works better than anything I've ever tried. It will take much longer to improve your form if you practice only during the first few minutes and then forget to do it for the remainder of your run.

PREPARING YOUR BODY

How many times have you gone out for a run and felt like your legs were made of concrete or worse? Well, I'll clue you in on a little secret: they might not feel so bad from something you *did* as from something you *didn't* do. Most people don't realize that taking good care of their body between runs is the best way to optimize the enjoyment and effectiveness of their workouts.

Here are some steps to take before going out for a run.

Eating

If you eat before you run, be sure it's at least three hours before. If you run in the morning, it's not really necessary to eat anything before you head out. Almost nothing you eat immediately before a run will be far enough into your system to help you during your run. If you do have to eat before running, be sure it's not a big meal, or you might end up with heartburn, stomachache, side stitches, or leaving it on the road somewhere. I've never heard of anyone starving to death on a run. In fact, if I'm hungry before I go running, it usually subsides within the first mile or two. It's best to run on an empty stomach, even on race days (with the exception of marathon distance or longer). Eating well the night before allows you to get up, get dressed, and head out in the morning. Then the biggest decision you might face is which route to follow.

Hydrating

If you run regularly, get yourself into the habit of drinking water all day long. It is recommended that the average person consume between 64 and 100 ounces of water daily, depending on a daily caloric expenditure of 2,000 to 3,000 calories. That's ten 10-ounce glasses of liquid. For the sake of your health, I'd suggest that it be mainly water, preferably filtered and not distilled. There are other forms of libation, but they all involve an increase in the work of your kidneys to filter out the extraneous ingredients. To keep from getting dehydrated, drink at least 8 ounces of water a half hour before heading out. If you're going longer than 5 or 6 miles, take along a water bottle or plan a route that has water stops along the way. Staying well hydrated will help your legs avoid cramping and keep your core body temperature within a reasonable range, especially in hot weather.

Body Looseners

Do not stretch before you run, stretching before you run can cause muscle pulls.

Instead do this set of Body Looseners before you head out the door. I call them "looseners" rather than "stretches" because they're meant to loosen your joints, not stretch your muscles. They're actually warm-up exercises for T'ai Chi, but if you do them religiously before you run, they will work wonders on the fluidity of your stride. If your joints are open and loose, your chi will flow through your body unhindered. Also, your muscles don't need to work as hard when your joints are loose. One of my longtime students has gotten so much benefit from these exercises that she now refuses to run unless she's done her looseners first.

This set of exercises is designed to loosen the main joint systems of the body, which are:

- Ankles
- Knees
- Hips
- Sacrum
- Spine
- Shoulders and neck

Exercise: Body Looseners

Begin by shaking out your lower legs and then your whole body. Let yourself get really floppy and loose.

- **Ankle rolls.** These will loosen all the ligaments and tendons in and around your ankles. Put your toes on the ground just behind your opposite foot. Keeping your toes on the ground, relax your ankle and rotate your knee in a circular motion to loosen your ankle. Do ten clockwise circles and then ten counterclockwise. Switch legs and repeat the exercise.
- **Knee circles.** This motion loosens the ligaments around your knees. Place your hands on your knees and move them around in small clockwise circles, then reverse the direction. Do ten in each direction.

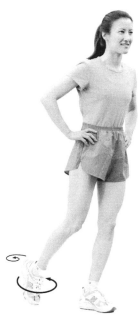

Figure 73—Ankle rolls

- **Hip circles** (figures 78 and 79). This exercise is easy to do but can be challenging to learn. It is, however, one of the best exercises there is for loosening your hips and pelvic area. Just take it slowly, and it'll come. I'll take you through it one step at a time. Stand up straight with your best posture stance, keeping your knees slightly bent. Keeping your feet flat on the ground, move your right knee in a circular clockwise direction. Do five "practice" circles, then return to your original stance. Next do five clockwise circles with your left

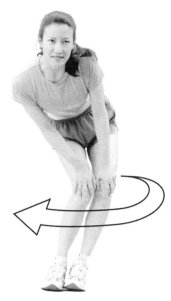

Figure 74—Knee circles to the left

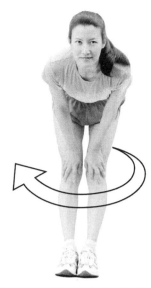

Figure 75—Knee circles to the back

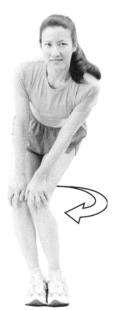

Figure 76—Knee circles to the right

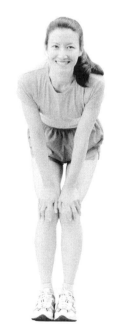

Figure 77—Knee circles to the front

knee. Now move *both* legs in a clockwise direction but a half cycle out of sync with each other (see figures 75 and 76). Start your knees going in circles by moving your right knee forward and your left knee back. This will get them each moving in their respective clockwise circles. If you start by moving your knees very slowly, it will come easier; you can always speed up as you get used to it. When they come back around to complete the circles, you will be in your starting position. Switch directions and repeat the exercise. Do ten circles in each direction. This exercise can be done anytime and anywhere, even when you're standing in line at the theater. Loosening this area will make your running very fluid and easy.

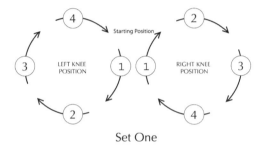

Set One

Figure 78—Hip circles

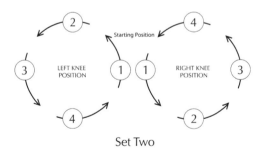

Set Two

Figure 79—Hip circles

- **Pelvic circles** (figures 80 to 83). This exercise loosens the area around your sacrum, which plays a key role in allowing you a relaxed leg swing. Place your hands on your hips, keep your back and spine in a vertical position, and tip your pelvis forward, to the side, to the back, to the opposite side, then back to forward. Do ten full circles with your pelvis and then change direction. When you get

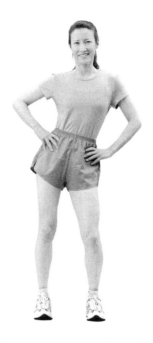

Figure 80—Hips to the right

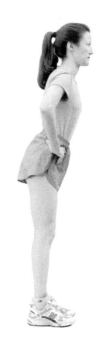

Figure 81—Hips to the back

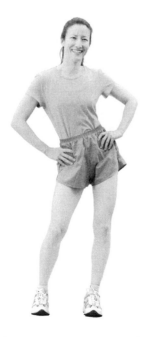

Figure 82—Hips to the left

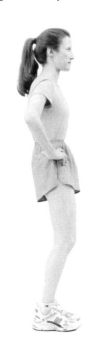

Figure 83—Hips to the front

smooth at this one, it will feel like you're belly dancing. Keep your upper body as motionless as possible as you make the circles with your pelvis.

- **Pelvic rotations** (figures 84 to 87). This exercise loosens your spine at T12/L1. Stand in a staggered stance with your arms held either straight out to your sides (like an airplane), or bent 90° at the elbow with the forearms pointed forward. Shift your weight forward with your front leg supporting 60% of your body weight and your rear leg supporting 40%. Keep both legs slightly bent at the knee. While holding your pelvis level, rotate it back and forth with as much range of motion as you can. Do twenty rotations, then shift your feet so that your opposite leg is forward and do twenty more.

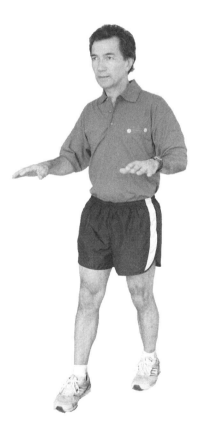 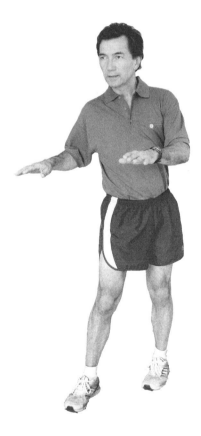

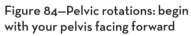

Figure 84—Pelvic rotations: begin with your pelvis facing forward

Figure 85—Rotate your pelvis to the left

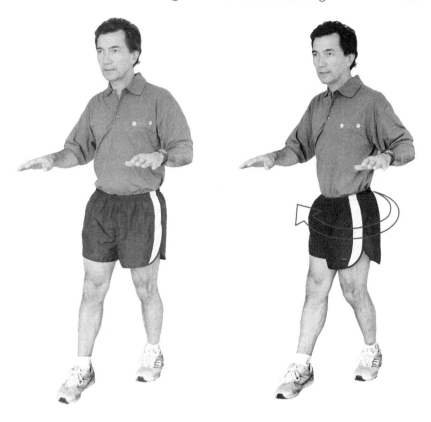

Figure 86—Rotate your pelvis back to forward

Figure 87—Rotate your pelvis to the right

Let *only* your lower body move during this exercise while your shoulders remain motionless.

- **Spine rolls** (figures 88 to 94). This exercise loosens all the ligaments along your spine. Stand up straight, place your hands on your upper thighs, and bend forward at the hips, keeping your spine as straight as possible. When you get as far over as your hamstrings allow, stretch your spine by pushing on your hips and lengthening the back of your neck at the same time. (This will loosen your spine by creating microspaces between each of the vertebrae.) Hold this stretch for five seconds, then soften your knees, flop over at the waist, and let your upper body just hang there upside down. Bend your knees slightly, and starting with your tail-

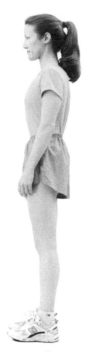

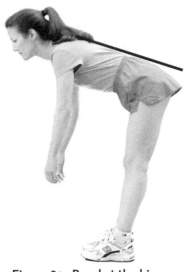

Figure 89—Bend at the hips and keep your back flat

Figure 88—Spine-roll starting position

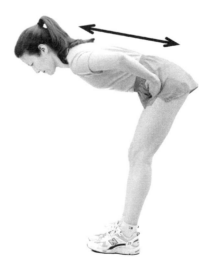

Figure 90—Stretch your spine in both

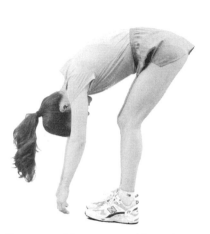

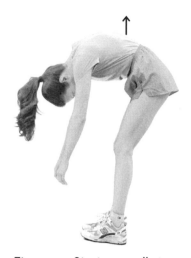

Figure 91—Flop over and hang limp

Figure 92—Start your roll at the lower back

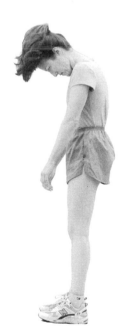

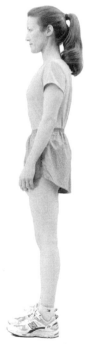

Figure 93—The last thing to lift is your head

Figure 94—Back to the starting position

bone, straighten yourself up one vertebra at a time until you are
vertical again. Do this very slowly. Repeat three times.

- **Spinal twist** (figures 95 to 98). This one loosens the tendons in
  your upper spine and shoulders, allowing you a relaxed arm swing.
  Stand with your feet together and your posture as upright as you
  can make it. Interlock your fingers behind your head with your elbows out to the side. Keeping your hips in a stationary position, rotate your upper body to the right. As you twist your upper body
  around, drop your right elbow and raise your left elbow so
  that your upper body is bent to the side. When you're
  twisted around, look down and try to see your opposite
  heel. Hold this position for a couple of seconds, then

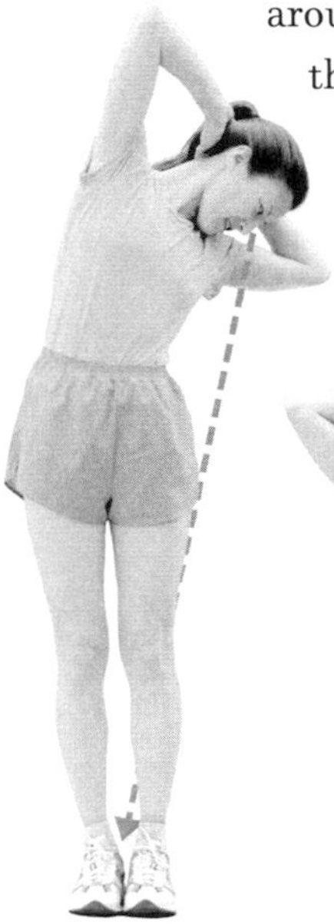

**Figure 95—Twist left
and look for your
opposite heel**

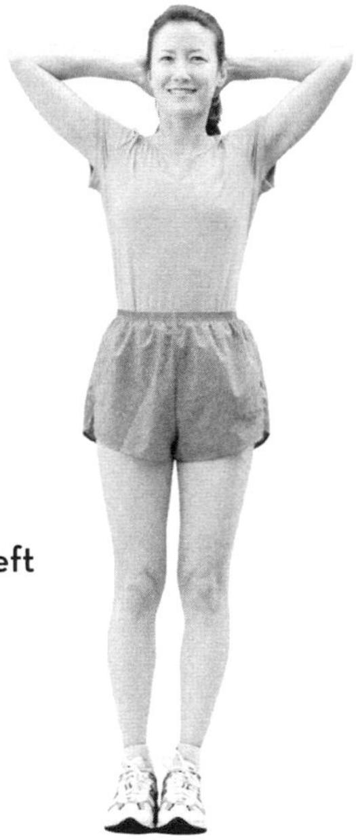

**Figure 96—Return to
the front**

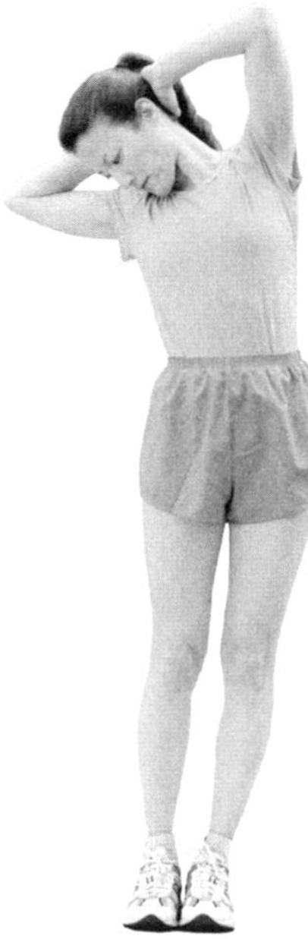

**Figure 97—Twist right
and look for your
opposite heel**

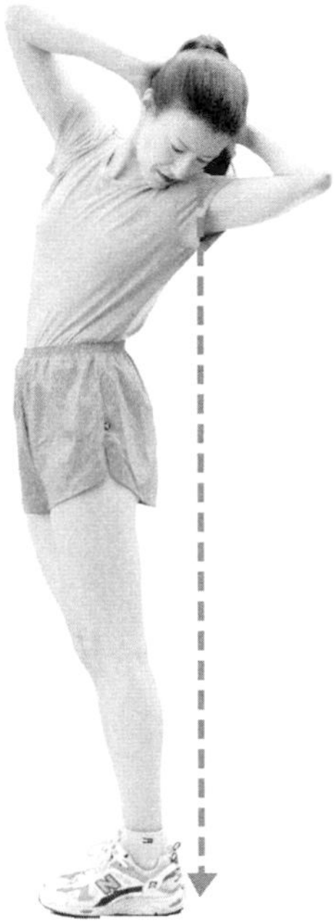

**Figure 98—Side view
showing line of sight**

come back to your starting position. Do the same thing on the left side. Repeat this exercise three times.

- **Shoulders and upper back.** Stand with your feet parallel and hip width apart. Then step straight back with one of your feet so the toe of that foot is lined up with the heel of the forward foot (as if you're starting a race), with your forward knee bent and your rear leg straight (figure 99). Lean your upper body out over your forward leg, keeping your spine straight. Now let your neck, arms, and shoulders totally relax while rotating your pelvis clockwise, then counterclockwise, like a washing machine (figure 100). Keep your arms and shoulders completely relaxed, and let them be swung by the rotation of your pelvis. Let your elbows bend as they swing behind your body so that the swinging motion won't pull on

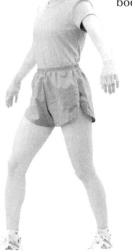

Figure 99—One foot behind the other: front leg bent, rear leg straight

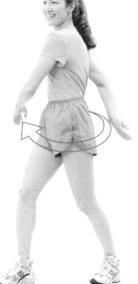

Figure 100—Use your hips to swing your shoulders

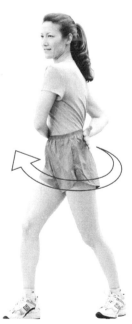

Figure 101—Bend your elbows

your shoulders (figure 101). Do
ten rotations then switch your
foot position and do ten more ro-

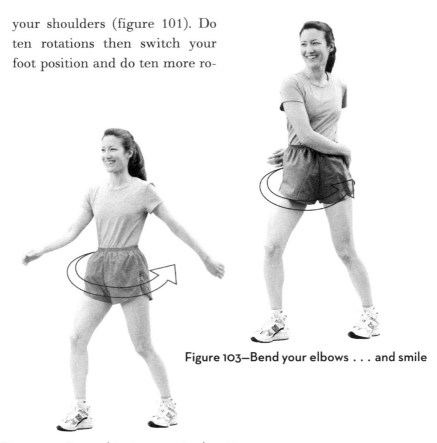

Figure 103—Bend your elbows . . . and smile

Figure 102—Rotate hips in opposite direction

tations. Now shake out your whole body and finish with the
grounding stance.

- **The Grounding Stance.** In ChiRunning, every foot strike is an opportunity to feel your feet on the ground and your structure supported by the earth. Do this exercise before every run to ground
  yourself in your body and feel the power of the earth beneath your
  feet.

  Stand upright with your best posture. Place your feet slightly
  wider than hip width apart. Soften your knees and let your arms
  hang at your sides. Feel your posture straight and tall. Focus your
  attention on your *dan tien* (your center, located three fingers below
  your navel). At the same time, drop your attention to the bottoms of
  your feet and press your big toes softly into the ground. Now con-

nect your *dan tien* to your feet with an imaginary line and let your feet support you. This will have the effect of rooting you to the earth. Hold this for at least thirty seconds. It'll feel like a long time, but it's worth every second if it leaves you feeling grounded. Master Xilin, my first T'ai Chi teacher, had me stand this way for the duration of our ninety-minute class—for weeks! He explained that it wouldn't do me any good to try to learn T'ai Chi if I couldn't feel grounded in my body first. Master Xu says it's one of the most difficult stances in T'ai Chi to master. I'm still working on it.

If you have access to one of those large stability balls, here's a great exercise to help get your body in the right alignment for the grounding stance. I call it the Chi-ball exercise.

1. Start by holding the ball in front of your body with your arms wrapped around it. Soften your knees and let the weight of your body sink into your feet (figure 104). Take a body snapshot of the position of your body and the physical sensations connected with it.

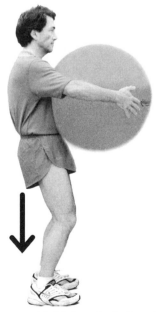 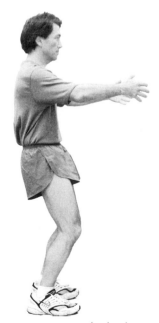

Figure 104—Hold the Chi-ball and sink   Figure 105—Remain in the body position

2. Now drop the ball while holding your body position (figure 105).

3. Next, relax your arms and let them fall to your sides without disturbing your body position. This is the grounding stance (figure 106).

4. Here's what the grounding stance looks like in motion (figure 107): subtract the left leg and tilt the runner upright, and there it is. In ChiRunning, every time your foot hits the ground, that's your grounding stance.

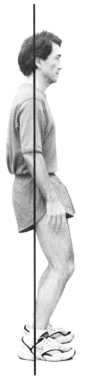 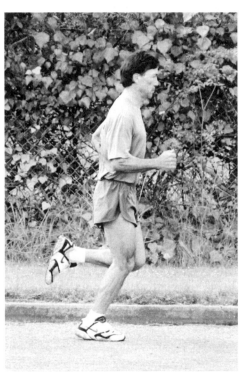

Figure 106—Grounding stance: shoulders, hips, and ankles aligned

Figure 107—The grounding stance in your stride

This set of looseners is a great pre-run ritual. Many ChiRunners make this a part of every workout.

TRANSITIONING OUT OF A RUN

You've just finished running. You're feeling pleasantly tired, and it's time to move on to your next activity. This is precisely the time to begin preparing for your next run. Sound crazy? Not so. In order for you to have a good run, whether it's tomorrow or the next day or next week, the best thing you can do for yourself is to treat your legs to a nice recovery so that when you run again, your legs will have a fresh start, with no carryover from the last session. If you take good care of your legs between runs, the quality of your next running session will be greatly enhanced.

Complementary to the pre-run themes of preparation and intention, the post-run themes change to recovery and assessment. After a run is the time to allow the results of your efforts to settle into your body and the time to do what it takes to physically recover so you can move into your next activity with a rejuvenated body and a clear mind. The mental aspect involves Body Sensing to assess how your run went: how it felt, what you learned, what worked and what didn't, and what you might do differently next time.

Here's a very enjoyable ritual for transitioning out of a run.

- **Ending a run.** If you just jump back in your car and head off to your next event you could end up walking around with tight legs. Give yourself a little time to switch out of running, and into the rest of your day. A cooldown and stretching period allows excess lactic acid to be flushed into your bloodstream and eliminated from your body. If it is allowed to linger in your system, studies show that it turns to concrete, or worse.
- **Cooling down.** When you cross your imaginary finish line, don't stop running. That's right, don't stop running, but reduce your speed to an effortless jog. This will allow your muscles to stay warm and help to circulate much of the metabolic waste out of your system. Take three to five minutes to jog at a very relaxed pace before slowing to a walk. Then take a few minutes to Body Sense how you feel. Let the run settle into your body. You should feel pleasantly

tired, not exhausted. Walk until your breath rate drops and your heart rate returns nearer to normal.

- **Stretching.** Even though I don't stretch before I run, I always stretch afterward. Here are a few injury-prevention guidelines for stretching. If you do it right, it will have an uncanny resemblance to yoga. Listen carefully to your body. I've seen too many people have great workouts and then pull a muscle while stretching. Never stretch a muscle until it hurts. Your stretches will be more effective if you take a soft and gentle approach. Relax and breathe out as you initiate each stretch. Hold each stretch gently for at least thirty seconds.

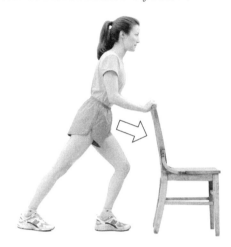

Figure 108—Calf/Achilles stretch

1. **Calf stretch.** Lean against a wall or chair with one heel extended on the ground behind you and the opposite foot on the ground at the base of the wall in front of you (figure 108). Move your pelvis toward the wall. This will stretch the calf muscles in your rear leg. Hold for a count of ten and repeat three times on each leg.

2. **Achilles stretch.** Same position, except you are dropping your rear knee down toward your forward heel. Hold for a count of ten and repeat three times on each leg.

3. **Hip flexor and upper hamstring stretch.** Rest one foot on top of a chair and move your pelvis toward the raised heel. Hold for a count of ten and repeat three times on each leg (figure 109).

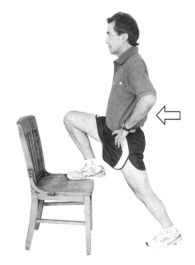

Figure 109—Hip flexor stretch

4. **Psoas stretch.** Stretches for the psoas are hard to come by, so I invented this one. If you have a tight psoas, you'll love it. Get into the same position as stretch #3, where your right foot is up on a chair and your left foot is on the ground. Take your left arm and hold it extended straight over your head with your *elbow locked* (figure 110). Now, move your pelvis in the direction of your elevated heel. This will stretch your hip flexor (as before). Stay in this position while sweeping

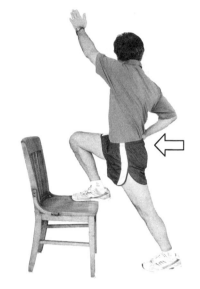

Figure 110—Psoas stretch: hip flexor stretch with upper body twist

your raised arm to the right as far as you can. Allow your body to bend sideways. To get the most amount of psoas stretch in this exercise it is crucial that you keep your elbow locked *at all times*. Hold the stretch for thirty seconds and then switch your leg position and do the same with your right arm sweeping to the left. Hold for thirty seconds.

5. **Hamstring stretch.** Place one heel on something hip height. Keeping both knees and your spine straight, bend your trunk toward your raised foot. Bend only as far as your hamstrings allow. Hold for a count of ten and repeat three times on each leg (figure 111).

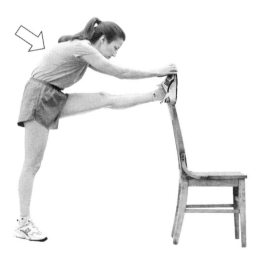

Figure 111—Hamstring stretch

6. **Adductor stretch.** Keeping your raised leg in position, turn your body 90° and let your upper foot rest on its side. With your spine straight, bend down to touch the toes of your support legs. This will stretch your adductors. Hold for a count of ten and repeat three times on each leg (figure 112).

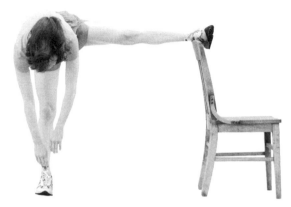

Figure 112—Adductor stretch

7. **Quadriceps stretch.** For this stretch, hold onto a chair with your free hand for stability. Or, for additional stretch, reach straight up over your head with your free hand. This move not only stretches your quads but builds the core muscles required for good balance. If you want to increase this stretch, hold this posture while picking up your pelvis in front. Hold for a count of ten and repeat three times on each leg (figure 113).

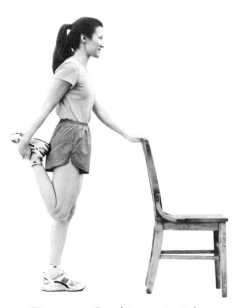

Figure 113—Quadriceps stretch

8. **Latissimus dorsi (lats) stretch.** This stretches the muscles of your lower back just below your shoulder blades. Stand vertical with your feet widely spread. Hold your arms horizontally out to your sides with your thumbs up. Tilt your upper body to one side until your arms make a vertical line, with one hand down and one hand up. Hold for a count of ten and repeat twice on each side. In yoga this is the triangle pose.

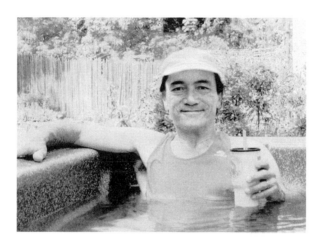

- **Soak your body.** If you have the luxury of being able to take a hot bath after your workout, do it. Soaking your legs warms your muscles and dilates your capillaries, which helps to flush metabolic waste out of your muscles and into your bloodstream to be eliminated. Hot baths have been one of my favorite rituals after running. And, given the hectic nature of our fast-paced world, I recommend hot baths whether you run or not.

  There seems to be a huge ongoing debate as to whether heat or cold is better for your legs after running. Cold is recommended if you have any inflammation, because it helps to reduce inflammation. But if you're not injured, cold doesn't make any sense, because it causes your muscles to contract, trapping some of the metabolic waste in your muscles. It's great to do a cold soak *after* a hot bath, or if there is *no* soreness in your legs after running. In fact, it feels very refreshing and allows your legs to feel revitalized as you move on to your next activity.

- **Leg drains.** When you're finished with your bath, do some "leg drains" by lying on your back with your feet propped up against a wall or chair (figure 115). Close your eyes and relax your entire body for three minutes. Then, using your hands, start at your ankles and squeeze down your legs toward your heart as if you're trying to wring the water out of a wet towel. This will allow the blood to drain out of your legs so that fresh clean blood can be pumped back in when you stand up. If your legs are not "cleaned out" after each run, you could start your next run with some of the "exhaust" from previous runs, which is no fun at all.

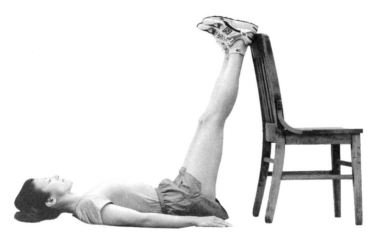

Figure 115—Leg drains

You can do leg drains either immediately after stretching or after your bath. Either way you'll notice a markedly different pair of legs under you when you get up. This is a great exercise to do anytime your legs feel tired. It's especially good for those of you who work on your feet. Try it. You'll be amazed.

- **Rehydrate.** Drink plenty of water after running. The rule that I use is "Drink before you get thirsty." If you finish a run with a dry mouth, your body is letting you know you didn't drink enough.

After your workout, drink small amounts until you're no longer thirsty. If you're tempted to grab a soft drink, just remember this: your kidneys are already stressed from doing overtime on the run, so it's a bit unfair to create more work for the poor little things by dumping in a bunch of chemicals and sugar. Stick to water or unsweetened fruit juice, and your kidneys will be happy as clams.

The more time you spend taking care of your body between runs, the more it will reward you with many years of enjoyable workouts. You'll also notice an increase in your performance level and the quality of your workouts.

THE POST-RUN MIND

I highly encourage an end-of-run review. The end of a run is another important time to practice Body Sensing and get as much post-run data from your body about your run as possible. Start by simply comparing how you felt at the beginning of the run to how you felt at the end.

I suggest keeping a running log. If you want to be really thorough, write in a journal.

Things to Track and Journalize

- Daily and weekly mileage
- Average pace on training runs
- Number of intervals and their relative split times (if done on the same course)
- Results of Body Sensing after a workout
- Aches and pains: location and intensity, what you were doing at the time
- Notable breakthroughs in your understanding of how your body is doing with the ChiRunning technique
- The age of your running shoes

The key word for transitioning into and out of your running is *mindfulness*. Being mindful during the time between runs will allow you to arrive at your next workout recovered and ready to be fully engaged. When you approach your running mindfully, each workout becomes more like a *living* ritual that leaves you with a sense of intention and depth.

By involving both your mind and body in your transitions, you will learn much more than good running skills. You'll develop qualities of thoughtfulness and presence that you can carry with you into the rest of your life. This approach to your running can help you live a life that is both focused and relaxed—two very useful qualities that *I'd* like to have when I grow up.

CHAPTER NINE

Troubleshooting: Injury Prevention and Recovery

We can't solve problems by using the same kind of thinking we used when we created them. —ALBERT EINSTEIN

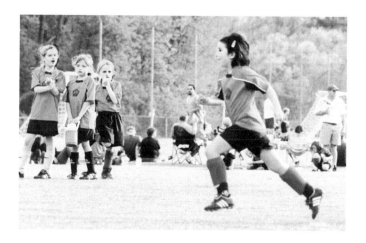

earning something new is the most powerful way to keep your body and mind vibrant. It's what gives life its spark, and it is what must take place in each of us if we hope to evolve as individuals. In any new undertaking, you can expect challenges—that's how you grow! Learning is always a stretch, which at times can feel uncomfortable physically, mentally, and emotionally. Use this chapter as a resource to guide you as you meet challenges such as injury or pain on the path to improving your running form.

It is crucial that you practice Body Sensing to become your own best authority over your body. We get thousands of e-mails from people asking if they can run with a particular injury or health condition. We also get letters from clients saying that their doctor has told them not to run. It is impossible for us to make these decisions for you. There *are* situations where you should no longer run. If running is threatening your long-term health in any way, then you should find another form of exercise, such as ChiWalking. However, there are many situations where if you correct how you are running you will no longer be hurting your body. What is most important is that you learn the ChiRunning form carefully. Take your time to make sure you are doing things correctly by using the DVD or working with a Certified ChiRunning Instructor. Then Body Sense, while running, the day after running, a few days after running, and over time. The skill of listening to your body and responding in the most appropriate and productive way, is always the best path.

Here is what Todd Toriscelli, head athletic trainer for the Tampa Bay Buccaneers, has to say about ChiRunning:

I have been an avid runner for well over twenty years. Like most runners, over time my pace slowed substantially, my exertion level increased, and I developed several consistent areas of pain throughout my body including my knees (three surgeries) and low back (multiple injections). I got to the point earlier this year that it just wasn't worth it anymore. As much as I loved running and competing in triathlons the pain and the poor performance associated with these events finally outweighed the benefits. I essentially decided to stop running, something I had enjoyed my whole life. A short time later, I was introduced to ChiRunning. As I read the philosophy behind it and about the technique it all made sense. I realized that my increase in pain and decrease in performance over the years was primarily due to an unsound running technique done to excess. It took its toll on my body.

Being a professional Certified Athletic Trainer, I deal with athletes on a daily basis and have good working knowledge of how the human body works. With this in mind, the more I learned about ChiRunning the more I realized that this is how a person should run. In some ways it contradicts what I have always thought about running and how to run. ChiRunning is a technique that requires reeducation. It is a hard concept to grasp for most of us, that running faster and with less effort doesn't involve increasing your muscle strength. It's all about technique and posture. Setting your body in the alignment of a Column, leaning forward, and allowing gravity to pull you forward instead of forcing your muscles to do the work is a much more efficient way to run. ChiRunning is a way to move in a natural, balanced way. As I took what I learned from the book and the DVD and started running, it was not easy to change. However, with time it is becoming more instinctive and natural. Since I started the technique my pain is gone and the enjoyment of running is back. My pace is quite a bit faster since I started, and according to my heartrate monitor less demanding on my body as a whole. ChiRunning in my opinion is truly a revolutionary approach to running and without question decreases the likelihood of injury.

THE DIFFERENCE BETWEEN PRODUCTIVE AND NONPRODUCTIVE DISCOMFORT

There's always some discomfort and awkwardness when you learn something new with your body. Do you know anyone who jumped on a bicycle for the first time and pedaled away without using training wheels first? Or anyone who stepped on a skateboard for the first time and didn't immediately fall right off? Learning is a process of trial and error, of trying and failing, of getting it and just as easily losing it. It can take a period of adjustment before everything moves along smoothly in the new way. During this period of transition, it is important to listen carefully to your body so you can tell whether or not you're moving correctly. One of the best ways your body has of telling you when you're doing something wrong is by sending your brain messages of discomfort or pain.

If there's any place in our culture where we need a healthy change in attitude, it's in our relationship with discomfort and pain. Instead of dealing with discomfort by addressing the cause, we are taught to deny its existence by using painkillers or some other course of symptomatic relief.

Since physical discomfort is a big issue with runners, I want to ease any fears around discomfort by clarifying the difference between productive discomfort and nonproductive discomfort. Productive discomfort leads to progress, while nonproductive discomfort leads to pain and/or injury (figure 117).

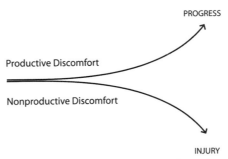

Figure 117—Productive and nonproductive discomfort

Productive discomfort is a necessary part of any growth process. For instance, when you start up a running program and get out of breath, it's uncomfortable to feel as if you're not getting enough air into your lungs. But it shouldn't come as any surprise that you breathe harder; after all, you're doing something that your body is not used to. If you can make it past the beginning stages, being out of breath will go away in a couple of weeks as your body acclimates to the increased oxygen requirements of running. Discomfort can be an indicator that you are going beyond your own status quo and feeling the stretch. Here are some everyday examples of productive discomfort:

- Headaches from quitting coffee
- Getting up earlier to exercise
- Feeling hungry because you're eating less to lose weight
- Running in inclement weather
- Feeling tired because of lack of sleep with a new baby
- Asking for a pay raise
- Standing in a five-hour line for Rolling Stones tickets

Another phrase used to describe productive discomfort was coined by the Russian mystic G. I. Gurdjieff, who called it "intentional suffering," which pretty much tells it like it is.

Nonproductive discomfort is a warning that something is not right with what you are doing, in which case you need to make an appropriate adjustment or the next sensation you might feel is pain. Pain is your body's way of telling you that you need to be careful not to let your situation degrade into an injury. Pain in your knees is an indication that you need to shorten your stride, land more on your midfoot, or correct an overpronation problem. Pain is your body's way of telling you to change how you're moving.

In my running career, I have learned the most about running correctly from pain. Whenever I've felt pain, I've had the choice to either stop running or to run in a way that prevented the pain from occurring. My first impulse has always been to look for the cause, which has inevitably led me to the solution. To make a correction to your running form, Body Sense precisely where the discomfort is coming from, so you have a point of reference from which to begin your correction.

Master Xu tells me that wherever you experience pain, your chi is blocked. If you can align, relax, and loosen the area that is painful, the chi will again flow through the area and help the pain to subside.

TRYING TOO HARD

You can most definitely try too hard when you are first learning the ChiRunning form. Gradual Progress is the watchword. We have found that people often lean too much or hold their posture too stiff. Trying to level your pelvis too much can lead to muscle soreness and pain. Wherever you feel pain in that part of your body, do the Body Looseners, relax, and have fun.

We've also had the "problem" of hearing that people are running faster than ever with less effort. Although this is in most cases a desirable result, we encourage runners to back off on their gas pedal, for safety reasons, until their body truly adapts to their new running form. Speed will happen. I spent many years doing long slow distance runs discovering the ChiRunning form. Many of our Certified ChiRunning Instructors are incredible runners, but they have all *learned* to run slowly to find the imperfections in their form and correct them at slow speeds, so that when they do go faster, their technique allows the speed to happen without injury.

COMMON RUNNING INJURIES

With a good working knowledge of what to do when things don't feel right, you can circumvent the difficulties or discomforts mentioned in the next section. This is a list of the most common concerns that we hear. Following the description of the symptom, I'll offer the likely causes, and in most cases I will refer you to the Form Focus most appropriate for your problem.

There is a plethora of books that deal with how to treat the *symptoms* of running injuries, so I won't go into that here. What I will say is that if you can work to correct the *cause* of a problem, you will increase your chances of the problem going away forever.

I will also say, as a disclaimer, that we are not licensed physicians, physical therapists, or health practitioners. All of the information contained in this section comes from twenty-five years of work done "in the field," helping thousands of people move past every running injury known. This information is based on the underlying movement and alignment principles of T'ai Chi, yoga, Pilates, the Alexander Technique, and the Feldenkrais Method, along with the latest thinking in the fields of sports physiology and biomechanics. For most running problems, we always recommend seeing a Certified ChiRunning Instructor. If you have an injury that is chronic or painful, see a trusted physical therapist, chiropractor, acupuncurist, or doctor. Your long-term health should be your top concern.

Use the following section as a reference if you feel any level of ache or pain.

Whenever you feel any discomfort, always try to ascertain its exact location. Then, go through this list of body topics and see if any of them fits your situation. Work with the recommended form correction and see if you can make a difference by changing something you're doing. Constantly Body Sense and "listen" to what your body has to say. Be patient with yourself and give yourself plenty of time to figure out a solution to your problem. If any of these suggestions works to alleviate your discomfort, remember to instate whatever focus you're using, before and during every run until the symptoms have disappeared.

For the sake of convenience, we've divided this section into three general categories: upper body, lower body, and general issues. To locate some of the muscles and tendons we talk about, see the Appendix.

In the following list you'll find the most commonly reported injuries from runners. There are a few areas of injury with which we have gone into an extended explanation of the symptoms, causes, and prevention/rehab tips. If you need further assistance and information about these injuries, please visit www.chirunning.com.

UPPER BODY

Neck Aches

Problems with your neck are generally due to your structure not being aligned properly, meaning that you need to work on correcting your posture (see figures 118 and 119). Neck pain can also be caused by holding your head in a stiff position with your chin held too far forward.

Breathing Issues or Shortness of Breath

The bottom line is that your muscles are not getting enough oxygen, and here are some possible reasons. Your breath may be too slow or too shallow, which means that your blood is not getting sufficiently oxygenated. You may also be running too fast for your current level of conditioning, or using too much muscle when you run. Go to Chapter 3 for a full explanation of issues around breathing.

Side Stitches

Here's my theory of what causes side stitches. Bear with me on this. Your organs are each suspended, surrounded, and held in place by a myofascial "sac" that attaches to the inside of your ribs. If you bounce when you run, it creates a tug on this attachment at the ribs, creating a sharp, localized pain. The two largest and heaviest organs in your trunk are your stomach (left-side stitch) and your liver (right-side stitch).

To get rid of either, here's what to do:

- **Practice running smoother along the ground.** Read the section on pelvic rotation, because it's the best way to keep from bouncing when you run.
- **For a right-side stitch,** using your thumb, find the space between the fifth and sixth ribs (counting from the lowest rib) on your right side, and rub it deeply and vigorously for thirty seconds. You'll know you have the right spot if it's really tender to the touch.
- **For a left-side stitch,** using your thumb, find the space between the fourth and fifth ribs (counting from the lowest rib) on your left side, and rub it deeply and vigorously for thirty seconds. Note that if you run too soon after eating, your stomach will weigh more and tug more on its attachment, giving you a side stitch on your left side.

Side stitches will also occur more often while running downhill because there is more tendency to bounce. If this is the case, shorten your stride, slow down your speed, and rub your ribs until the discomfort goes away.

Shoulder Aches

Many people who complain of tight shoulders tend to run with their shoulders held either too far back or too high. Here are some suggestions:

- **If you hold your shoulders too high, relax them** by dangling your arms at your sides for one minute every fifteen minutes while you're running. To reestablish your arm swing, bend your arms at a right angle and focus on your *elbows* swinging rearward, keeping your shoulders relaxed and low. They should feel the same as when you were dangling your arms. Focusing on the elbows makes a huge difference.
- **Don't use your shoulders to swing your arms.** Let your arms swing on their own.

- **If you work at a desk job, take hourly breaks** from sitting down. Stand up, breathe deeply, do a few shoulder rolls, and lower your shoulders often.
- **Doing the "C" shape repeatedly** will also help you to relax your shoulders.

Upper Back

Upper back pain can happen if you have a slumped or round-shouldered posture and then take on the work of straightening up your posture. Lengthen the back of your neck while dropping your shoulders at the same time, while running *and* throughout your day.

Chest Pain

This is one discomfort you definitely *don't* want to have when you're running. If you ever experience any dull or sharp chest pain, it could be an indication of heart problems. Stop your run immediately and ask for assistance from anyone nearby. Do not start up your run again, even if the pain goes away. You're done for the day. Consult your doctor as soon as possible.

LOWER BODY
Lower Back

Having tightness or soreness in your lower back can mean that you're bending at the waist as you land on your support leg instead of keeping your pelvis level and your posture straight. Bending at the waist forces your lower back muscles to support the weight of your upper body, because it's cantilevered in front of you (figure 118). Running with straight posture allows

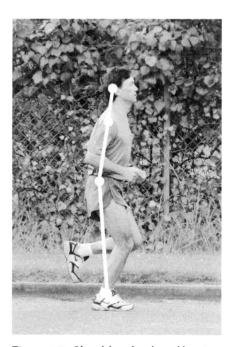

Figure 118—Shoulders back and bent at the waist

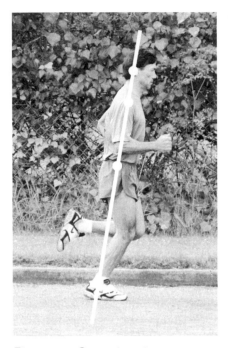

Figure 119—Correct posture: ear, shoulder, hip, and ankle aligned

your structure to support your body weight, as it should (figure 119). Do the "C" shape often. Use your abdominal muscles to support your posture, and your back muscles will not be overworked.

Hip Joints

Hip pain can be a symptom of many different issues, but generally speaking it's from tension in your hips. Loosen 'em up, baby! Do hip circles (see page 196) all day, every day.

Hip pain can also be caused by a lack of core strength. When you have too little core strength to stabilize your pelvis while running, your hips will move laterally, causing your pelvis to sway side to side and your hip joints to bend in a direction it was not designed to. This will irritate either the bursa or the IT band and show up as hip pain. If you have hip pain, practice leveling your pelvis whenever you're walking, running, or standing, as this will stabilize your pelvis, and keep your hips in the best alignment for supporting your body weight. It sounds simple, but it'll work wonders on your sore hips.

Groin Pulls

This is an injury that can make the simple act of swinging your legs much more painful and difficult than you can imagine. The runners who get groin pulls are, generally speaking, those whose feet splay out to some extent while running (see page 66, figures 9 and 10).

Hip Flexors

This muscle group lifts your leg either upward (picking up your knees) or forward (returning your leg to the support phase). When it's sore, it's an indication that you're overdoing one or the other. Lifting your knees, as we have mentioned, is not only inefficient, it can cause you to overstride. Returning your leg to the support phase does not require you to use the hip flexors in an active way; instead, allow the recoil of the hip flexor tendon to return your leg to its resting position. When your leg swings out behind you, the hip flexor tendons are stretched like a rubber band. As soon as your foot leaves the ground, the recoil of the tendons will return your leg to the midfoot strike position. Because of the recoil action of the tendons, your hip flexors don't need to "work" to accomplish this. The best remedy for sore hip flexors is to rotate your pelvis more as you run.

Quadriceps

If your quads are sore, it means you're using them too much. Sorry, overuse is not allowed in ChiRunning. Generally, if your quads hurt, it means that either your foot is striking in front of your body or you're bending at the waist (and most likely both). Doing either of these increases the impact to your upper legs. Shorten your stride and pull your foot strike back in, so you're landing in a midfoot strike, and you'll reduce the shock to your quads.

Hamstrings

Most people feel hamstring pulls at the top end where the hamstrings attach to your pelvis, just under your glutes. This is usually experienced as a burning sensation. If this is going on for you, it's generally because your foot is striking in front of you and you're overstriding, pulling yourself forward with each step. This puts an inordinate amount of responsibility onto your hamstrings since they were not "designed" to do this much work. It also happens when you're running uphill and reaching ahead of your body with your legs. Let your lean do the work so your upper body is ahead of where your feet are striking the ground, and the pulling will disappear (see Chapter 7). Keep your feet from striking ahead of your hips.

Glutes

Any pain felt in your glutes is generally from tension held there. If you feel tightness or soreness in your glutes, it's your body telling you that you're a tight-ass, just like the rest of us who hold tension there. This is not "Buns of Steel" class, so you've got to learn to relax and let energy flow through that area.

If you can relax here, you can relax anywhere. If you hold tension here, it usually means you have to work on your control issues. Go ahead and let go. Your friends will love you for it.

Iliotibial Band Syndrome

You might have also heard this referred to as ITB syndrome. This is one of the most common injuries experienced by runners and walkers alike. It's a painful tightening along the outside of the thigh that can bring your run or walk to a halt if left unchecked. This is such a common injury that we give a very thorough explanation here.

The iliotibial band is a thick fibrous band running along the outside of the leg from the hip (ilium) to the shin bone (tibia) just below the kneecap—like a stripe down the side of your leg. In the hip area the upper end of the IT band and the hip are joined together by a muscle (the tensor fascia latae), which you can see just under the shorts on many lean runners and walkers. The IT band's job is to hold the upper and lower parts of your leg stable when your knee bends. Specifically, it works in partnership with the muscles on the inside of your thigh to keep your knee from collapsing inward on every step.

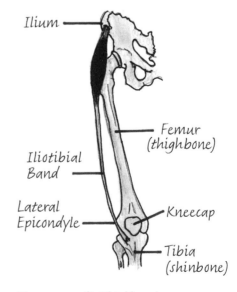

Figure 120—Iliotibial band

ITB syndrome is a repetitive use injury that occurs when the band tightens up, often because of too much side-to-side rocking of the hip. As the band tightens up, each step can pull it tighter across the bones of the knee joint and actually rub on the outer part of the knee.

This rubbing can cause inflammation and pain, usually around the outside of the knee. You may or may not see swelling, but the pain can be enough to stop you in your tracks. Even if you don't experience knee pain, the band may be tight enough to be tender all along the outside of your thigh. Often the pain may not appear until you are a mile or two into your workout, and may feel worse as you continue or when you run or walk downhill or downstairs. Many times the pain will subside if you stop running momentarily and walk with very short steps. That's because walking minimizes the rubbing of the band over the joint. Most often IT band problems occur at the knee, but you may also feel discomfort closer to your hip, and/or all along the IT band due to its tightness.

One of the most common causes of IT band soreness happens in runners and walkers whose pelvis sways side to side with each step. (An exaggeration of this motion would be a fashion model walking down a runway.) Any lateral (sideways) movement of your pelvis will tighten your IT band because as your foot lands under you, your hip moves sideways. This not only overstretches the IT band, making it sore, but can also aggravate the bursa of the hip, creating hip bursitis.

Another common cause of IT band tightness is running or walking with your toes pointed outward. This causes the foot to overpronate or roll inward excessively as your heel strikes the ground, making the IT band work harder to control the inward motion. Any tightness in your leg muscles can make IT band symptoms worse, and symptoms may also appear after ramping up your mileage too quickly.

Here's what you can do about it:

- **Focus on keeping your pelvis level,** front to back and side to side. This will solve most IT band problems. Level your pelvis in between runs as well.
- **Apply ice and massage.** If your IT band area is so sore that every

step hurts no matter what, you may want to help it out in between runs by icing the inflamed area or by massaging the entire IT band. A foam roller does a nice job of this. This may hurt a little, but it will really help. Lie on your side with the outside of the affected leg on the foam roller about halfway down the thigh; roll up and down until you find a sore spot, then stop and rest on that spot until the pain reduces by about 75%—it takes a few seconds. Breathe. Move to the next tight spot and repeat. Do this on both sides, even if you don't have IT band soreness in both legs.

- **Shorten your runs or walks** while you are recovering. If you run or walk at the track, change your direction often or do your intervals sets counterclockwise and your recoveries the other way.

Knees

By far the most complaints I get from runners is that running is so hard on their knees. Secretly, I have my own complaint about running that is a little different. It's that running is blamed for all the knee problems when in actuality it's not the running that is causing the injuries, but the way people run. Every time someone's knee goes out and their friends ask them how it happened, they're quick to respond, "It happened the other day while I was running." The truth is that if you can improve your running technique so that there is minimal impact or undue stress to your knees, you'll never have knee problems. It's that simple.

Here are some ways to protect those precious knees and ensure that you can run for many more years without the worry of having to give it all up someday because your knees are toasted.

- **Don't heel strike.** Land in a midfoot strike and don't let your feet land ahead of you. Always lean from your ankles and let your stride open up *behind* you so that when your legs swing forward, your feet don't land in front of you, but underneath or slightly behind your center of mass.
- **Don't pick up your knees when you run.** That's right. Pay no attention to the advice of all those running magazines that tell you to pick up your knees and reach forward for a longer stride. When you

lift your knees, your lower leg will swing forward and your heel will hit with a braking motion in front of your body.

Keep your knees swinging low. At the back end of each stride, keep your knees low and let your heels float up behind you. You should always be thinking, "Knees down . . . heels up."

- **Keep your knees soft and bent** during the landing and support phases of your stride. I see many runners overstride and then straighten their knees when they land. This creates an incredible amount of impact to the heel and the knee.

- **Foot turnout.** If your feet splay out to the side as you run, it could create knee pain while running any distance because you're twisting your knee with every foot strike. This will eventually over-stretch the medial ligaments and tendons of the knee and lead to pain and/or injury (medial meniscus tendonitis). You'll feel it as a sharp pain on the inside (medial side) of your knee.

Here's what happens. If your feet splay out with every step, you'll land on the outside edge of your heel and your ankle will collapse inward. This creates a torque in your lower leg that is the equivalent of someone grabbing your ankle and twisting it to the outside 85–90 times every minute! It doesn't take very many miles of running this way for your knees to start feeling the stress.

Learn to run with your feet pointed in the direction you're headed. To do this, rotate your entire leg inward toward your centerline until your feet are parallel and pointing forward. This will strengthen your adductors (the muscles that run along your inner thighs) and straighten out your legs. This allows your knees to hinge in the direction they were designed to, instead of twisting with each footstep.

Running with your feet turned out can also aggravate the iliotibial band, which is attached at its lower end to the lateral side of your tibia just below your knee. See "Iliotibial Band Syndrome" (page 228).

Taking good care of your knees should be a high priority, especially if you want to continue to enjoy running year after year. Reducing torque and impact are the two best places to build a life insurance policy for your knees. Start today and your knees will thank you every time you put on your running shoes.

Shin Splints

There are very few runners I've come across that haven't at some point in their running career had a case of shin splints, varying in degree from mild shin pain to a debilitating stress fracture of the tibia. But although it is one of the most common injuries known to runners, it is easily curable and preventable. Here's how you can avoid having shin splints for the rest of your life.

"Shin splints" is sort of a catchall phrase for a number of ailments that occur in the lower leg. The medical name for shin splints is medial tibial stress syndrome (MTSS). In the mildest cases, shin splints are the inflammation of the fascia (connective tissue) that covers and connects the muscles of the lower leg to the bone (the tibia). In the worst case, the fascia is under such stress that it actually separates from the tibia, which is very painful and can involve a rather slow healing process.

Shin splints can happen in a variety of ways. Here are a few:

- **Dorsiflexing your ankles as your legs swing forward.** When you dorsiflex your ankles, it means that you pick up your toes as you swing your feet forward. I think I can safely say that well over 60% of all runners dorsiflex with every stride. When you dorsiflex, you're contracting your shin muscle (tibialis anterior). As your heel hits the ground, it acts as a fulcrum, your toes slam down into the ground, and the sudden extension of your ankle pulls against the contracted shin muscle. If done repeatedly (as in downhill running or overstriding), the fascia that connects your shin muscle to the bone can actually get pulled loose from the bone and inflamed.
- **Heel striking.** To avoid shin splints, it is important to eliminate any heel strike while running (see the section on the lean in Chapter 4).
- **Running on your forefeet.** Running on your forefeet or pushing off with your toes causes the calf and shin muscles to overwork.

Anytime your body weight is supported by your toes, your calves and shins are required to do much more work than they were designed to do (figure 122).

- **Downhill running.** Many people get shin splints from running downhill. This happens because as you go downhill there is a need to put on the brakes to slow yourself and maintain a safe speed. Unfortunately, we all tend to land on our heels (by dorsiflexing) as a means of putting on the brakes.
- **Running farther or faster than your body is ready to.** Beginning runners who are starting up a running program will often run too far or too fast before their legs are ready to sustain the distance or the speed they're running. Add to this the fact that almost all beginning runners push off with their toes, which increases the stress to their unconditioned legs, especially the shins.

Eliminate Shin Splints Forever!

The pain of your shin splints might go away with rest, but as soon as you get back on your feet running again, you might notice the same old problem coming back to haunt you. If this is the case, you have a couple of options from which to choose. One option is to gradually strengthen the muscles in your lower legs by doing such things as calf raises or walking on your heels. This will sometimes work, but it is not necessarily a guaranteed way to permanently rid yourself of shin splints. Remember, it is not your shins that create shin splints. It's the way you run.

- **Reduce or eliminate the use of your lower legs while running.** You can heal or greatly reduce your odds of getting shin splints this way. Since gravity is your main source of forward propulsion, in ChiRunning your shin muscles are not engaged. This takes almost all of the work off the shins because they are only needed for momentary support between strides.
- **Keep your lower legs relaxed at all times,** allowing your foot to *land in a midfoot strike*, slightly behind your center of mass. *Keep your shin muscles relaxed* and you'll eliminate any chance of landing with your ankle dorsiflexed.

- **Practice the Sand Pit Exercise regularly** if you have shin splints (see page 133).

With practice, you can learn to run without ever overworking your lower legs, and put the threat of shin splints out of your mind and body forever. Think of your lower legs this way: if you don't use them, you can't abuse them. Keep them relaxed whenever you're running or walking, and your running future will look (and feel) a lot rosier.

Calf Pulls and Soreness

If your calves are sore, it's because you're using them, which is counter-indicated for ChiRunners. Practice relaxing them and try to always land in a midfoot strike (see figure 121). Talk to your calves and ankles. Tell them you're going out for a run and they have the day off.

- **Be sure you're not leaning too far forward** and engaging your lower legs to hold your angle of lean (see "window of lean" example in Chapter 4, page 84).

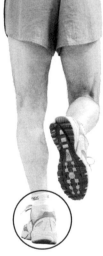

Figure 121—Landing on the midfoot (correct)

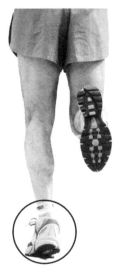

Figure 122—Up on the balls of the feet (incorrect)

- **Keep your legs limp from the knees down** as a constant, ongoing practice whenever you're walking or running. A client once told me that he remembered to keep his lower legs limp by pretending he didn't have any lower legs.
- **Practice peeling up your feet** while keeping your legs limp from the knees down, and give yourself the goal of mastering the Sand Pit Exercise (see page 89).
- **Shake out your lower legs often** whenever you're standing around. Teach them to relax! Practice relaxing your calves at all times, not just when you run, but whenever you're walking too.
- **If you're recovering from calf pulls, be sure to run on flat surfaces.** Running up hills will sometimes force you onto your toes, which will aggravate your calves.
- **Be sure you are landing on your midfoot** (which engages your core muscles) and not on the ball of your foot (which engages your calves) (figures 121 and 122).
- **If your calves are chronically tight, massage them often**, especially after each run. Constantly work at not holding tension in your ankles, and take hot baths after workouts.
- **Make sure to take in enough water or electrolytes while running**. Not doing so cramps the calves, which can be very painful and can quickly reduce a run to a walk. Also, remember that if you don't overuse your calves, they'll never be starved for electrolytes.
- **Shorten your stride.** If it is too long, it will engage your calf muscles as your foot leaves the ground.
- **Check to see if your shoes are too stiff.** They should be very flexible in the forefoot. If they're not, it will cause you to engage your calf muscles needlessly.
- **Look at the bottoms of your shoes to see the wear patterns.** If your shoes are worn at the toe, you're pushing off. If they're worn at the heel, you're heel striking, which means that your stride is too long and that you're reaching with your forward leg.
- **Stretch the calf and Achilles tendon**. Stand on a curb facing away from the street with the midfoot of the sore foot resting on the edge of the curb and your heel extending out beyond the curb, keeping the healthy foot completely on the sidewalk for stability.

Then slowly lower your heel enough to give your Achilles tendon and calf muscle a good stretch. Hold this for twenty to thirty seconds and repeat three times.

Muscle Cramps

These are caused mostly by dehydration and/or a low level of electrolytes. If your body is low on water or electrolytes, it will have a difficult time conducting the electrical current necessary for the firing of your muscles. For prevention, drink 12 ounces of water or sports drink a half hour before you exercise. If you'll be out running for more than an hour, carry your own water or sports drink. Test out various sports drinks on your runs to see how your body adapts to each one. Look for one that is easy to drink, tastes decent, and doesn't have an ingredients label that looks like a chemistry final.

When I'm racing, I set my countdown timer for ten-minute intervals and drink electrolyte replacement fluid every time it goes off. This keeps me well hydrated, and I never have muscle cramps. I call it the drip system. An alternative to electrolyte replacement drinks is taking electrolyte capsules (not salt tablets). They eliminate the need to carry anything except water. And the best part is that you don't have to drink that nasty stuff they serve at aid stations. (See Chapter 10 on race training.)

Achilles Tendonitis

You'll begin to feel Achilles tendonitis as a burning sensation just above your heel. Relax your entire lower legs when you run, and your Achilles tendons will never be overworked.

- **Run on soft, flat surfaces** until the soreness is gone. When you add hills back into your program, just make them light and easy at first.
- **Run slowly** and don't increase your speed during workouts unless your Achilles tendon says it's okay to do so.
- **Don't stop walking or running, although you might be tempted** when you have an Achilles pull. Without some amount of stretching during the healing process, it will heal at a shorter length, leaving you vulnerable to a repeat injury. Just shorten your stride and walk or run at a slower pace.

- If it's just too painful to run on, take it easy and run at the first possible opportunity. Ice it often to keep any swelling down. Achilles tendon pulls are one of the best times to learn how to relax your lower legs when you run and walk.
- Pool running is a great way to keep your legs in shape while recovering from an Achilles pull.

Plantar Fasciitis

There are a few things in this world I would not wish on my worst enemy. Plantar fasciitis (PF, pronounced "fah-shee-*eye*-tiss") is one of them. If you've ever had it, you know what I mean. When I feel it coming on, I get a sensation in my gut similar to what Harry Potter felt when he knew the Death Eaters were after him—I'll do anything in my power to guard against it becoming a full-blown reality.

This debilitating (not to mention annoyingly persistent) injury can happen to runners and walkers alike. And it's harder to get rid of than a condo in a recession. I've had my bouts with it and I'd like to offer anything I can to those of you who either wish to recover from PF or avoid it altogether.

The plantar tendon runs the length of the bottom of your foot, spanning the area from the base of the toes to the front of your heel. If you think of the arch of your foot as a bow (as in bow and arrow), imagine the plantar tendon as the bowstring. The two ends of the bowstring attach at the base of the toes and at the front of the heel bone by means of fascia, a strong fibrous membrane. The bowstring (plantar tendon) keeps the arch of the foot from flattening completely when the foot is bearing weight, thus providing cushioning and shock absorption when you're walking, running, or standing (see figure 123). This tendon also allows you to point your toes.

PF is an inflammation

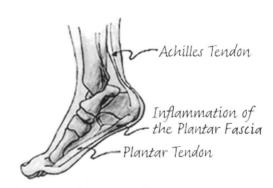

Figure 123—Plantar tendon

of the plantar fascia where it connects the plantar tendon to either the heel bone or to the base of the toes. It can be caused by any motion of your legs that creates a pull or impact to the plantar tendon. That means walking or running up or down hills, climbing stairs, walking or running on your toes (yes, that includes wearing high heels), or dorsiflexing.

It can also be caused by heel striking while overstriding or running downhill. If you're reaching forward with your legs (see figure 51, page 107) with each stride, you're very likely to land on your heel, which can create a force on your heels of up to six times your body weight with each footstep. That is a very small area to be absorbing that much impact. The surface area of your heel is about 2 square inches. If you weigh 125 pounds and you're running with a heel strike, that means the force to your heel is, conservatively, 250 pounds per square inch of force on your heel with each stride. With that kind of pressure, it's no wonder you end up bruising the spot where the plantar tendon attaches to the heel.

Here's another way you might end up with PF. On the rear side of your heel is the attachment of the Achilles tendon, which runs up into your calf muscle. If your calves are tight and/or your Achilles tendon is not flexible, you will be pulling and tightening the plantar tendon and weakening the attachment of the fascia to the bone. If for some reason the plantar tendon is pulled beyond what the fascia is capable of holding, the fascia forms microtears and begins to pull away from the bone. This causes the fascia to become inflamed (fasciitis).

Here's a long-term situation to avoid. If the plantar tendon is consistently overstretched for weeks or months, the body begins to add calcium where the attachment between the tendon and the heel bone takes place. Over time enough calcium is added to actually build more bone mass in that particular spot on the heel, and you end up with a heel spur, which is even more painful than PF. Imagine feeling pain every time you take a step and feeling pain thousands of times every day. No thanks. I'll do whatever I can to avoid that.

Other causes of PF are:

- Inflexible shoes, worn-out shoes, or shoes that bend in the middle instead of the ball of the foot
- Low arches or high arches
- Being overweight
- Spending long hours on your feet
- Walking barefoot in soft sand for long distances if your feet are not used to it

What does PF feel like? Of course this is a very subjective question so I'll try to give you a range of sensations, progressing from nuisance to agony. When PF first appears it can feel like you've got a lump in the heel of your sock. No big deal, no pain . . . just an uncomfortable "thick" feeling right under your heel. I find myself taking out the insole to my shoe to see if there's maybe a rock trapped underneath. If, after replacing the insole and straightening my sock out, I still feel a lump under my heal, I take it very seriously. The Death Eaters are on their way if I don't do something!

When you feel this, you know that you've slipped into some old habits and that you need to practice landing with a midfoot strike. This will insure that your ankles remain relaxed and your plantar tendon is not overstretched.

In the next level of PF your heel will feel a little tender when you first get up from a chair or get out of bed in the morning. In the early stages the discomfort will go away once you're up and about on your feet. But as the injury advances into later stages, the tenderness will linger and begin to turn into what feels like little needles sticking you in the bottom of your heel with each step. Trust me, it's not fun.

In the very advanced stages of PF, you find yourself surfing Amazon to find books on levitation. It aches all day, not just when you're walking or running.

I think I can safely say there's no instant cure for PF, except for maybe divine intervention. Believe me, I've wished many times there were. It takes time for the inflammation in the fascia to subside and to heal any tears in either the tendon or the fascia. In fact, right up front, when you feel the first symptoms of PF, I suggest you make an agreement with yourself that *you* will be more persistent than *it*. Any injury like this is a great opportunity to practice mindfulness in your movement. Be as consistent as possible with all of your ChiRunning Form Focuses to stave off PF, as it can take quite a while to heal.

Here are some steps you can take at the first indication of soreness in your heel.

- **Learn to relax your lower legs,** especially your ankles and calves, whenever you're walking, running, sitting or standing. Tension held anywhere in your legs or glutes will pull on the plantar tendon when you move. Relax, relax, relax, or suffer the consequences.
- **Always be mindful of landing with a midfoot strike when running.** Never strike on the back of your heels.
- **Don't reach forward with your legs when running.** Let your upper body lead and let your legs follow. This will help you maintain a midfoot strike and avoid all that pounding to your heel. . . . one of the biggest culprits in PF.

Additional things to do:

- **Shorten your stride length** when walking or running.
- **Walk and run on soft, flat surfaces** as much as possible. Avoid hills, trails, and uneven surfaces.
- **Avoid stairs**—treat yourself to an elevator.
- **Improve the flexibility** of the calf muscles and Achilles tendon which pull on the plantar tendon. (See "Strengthening and Stretching the Feet" exercises beginning on page 242.)
- **Get a foot massage,** the deeper the better.

Treatment if you are in acute pain:

- **Soak your heel in a big bowl of ice water** (five to ten minutes) twice daily until the pain subsides. It's excruciating but well worth it.
- **If you do drugs, take ibuprofen** for treating inflammation, but PF can last a long time and you should not take ibuprofen too often.

- **Orthotics** can help reduce the pain on the bottom of the heel, but be mindful that they will not fix the reason why you have PF. If you don't want to be tied to orthotics for months or years, you'll need to change your movement habits, which are causing the problem.
- **Do more stretches and strengthening exercises,** see "General Advice on the Feet and Ankles." All of this should set you well on your way to either preventing PF or gradually ridding yourself of this all-too-common but avoidable problem. With this particular injury there's an old saying that absolutely pertains: "An ounce of prevention is worth a pound of cure."
- **Walk on a coarse gravel surface:** This can be done barefoot or in stocking feet. Again, those of you with plantar fasciitis will "love" this one. It hurts, but it gets rid of PF faster than anything else I've ever tried. Do it for ten minutes a day until the symptoms disappear.

GENERAL ADVICE ON THE FEET AND ANKLES

Each of your feet has twenty-six bones, thirty-three joints, and more than a hundred muscles, ligaments, and tendons. In addition to that, your feet are responsible for supporting your entire body weight, no matter how you're moving. That's a lot of small parts that need to keep up with a huge responsibility. It's no wonder that there are so many things that can go wrong with your feet, especially if anything upstairs is moving either incorrectly, inefficiently, or in an imbalanced state. It all comes down to the feet, because that, as they say, is where the rubber meets the road. In T'ai Chi, your connection with the earth is paramount to all else, because if you lose that connection you'll never be able to stand up against any opponent, because you won't feel the flow of chi from the earth, filling your body with powerful energy.

Besides supporting your body, your feet serve in another, equally important capacity. From infancy, our feet teach our bodies how to move. From the time we first learn to stand and walk, all of our balance and movement is dependent on the messages being sent to our brain from our feet. If this messaging system is altered in any way, our brain won't get a clear message of how to move our body correctly. This is one reason why many physical therapists nowadays are having their clients walk barefoot in order to reeducate their bodies into correct movement patterns after an injury. It's also the reason why I believe the Kenyans and other East Africans are such beautiful runners. It's because they spend many more years of their lives running barefoot than we do. And because of this, I've never seen a Kenyan with a heel strike. It doesn't happen. Similarly with children—when I watch my daughter run down the street barefoot, I see a beautiful forward lean, a perfect midfoot strike, and her legs flying out behind her. There's nothing I could, or would, correct.

Our feet and ankles need to be strong yet flexible in order to do their job. If they're too weak or rigid in any way, problems begin to occur. So the best thing you can do for your feet is take very good care of them, and there are two basic ways to accomplish this: through exercises designed to flex and strengthen your ankles and feet, and by wearing shoes that allow your feet all the freedom they need to do their job well and as naturally as possible.

Here are some things you can do to strengthen the muscles and tendons in your feet and ankles, along with some suggestions for keeping them supple and flexible.

Exercise: Strengthening and Stretching the Feet

- **Ankle-strengthening exercise.** Here's a great exercise for strengthening the medial muscles, tendons, and ligaments in your ankles and legs. This exercise will not only add stability to your ankles but also strengthen your arches. This is a great exercise for people with flat feet, overpronators, people whose feet splay out, and those with bunions on the medial side of the big toe.
  1. Lie on your back with your feet together and your legs extended.
  2. Prop yourself up onto your elbows, leaving your lower back in contact with the floor.
  3. Contract your lower abdominal muscles and level your pelvis by pressing your lower back into the floor and holding it there.
  4. Lock your knees while dorsiflexing your ankles (point your toes toward your head).

5. Here's the last but most important part of this exercise: while doing all of the above, touch your big toes together and rotate your ankles as if you're trying to touch the bottoms of your feet together. You should feel every muscle and tendon on the medial side of your legs contract.

6. Hold this position as long as you can and then let go and relax your whole body by just lying on the floor. Repeat after a ten-second break. Do at least five of these every day as a regular habit. Strengthening these muscles and tendons takes consistent work over a long period of time (sometimes years) in order to show change. But if you can stick with it for the duration, you can rid yourself of any problems associated with any of the maladies mentioned at the beginning of this exercise.

- **Ankle rolls.** These are great for loosening all the muscles and tendons of the ankle. They're described in the section on Body Looseners (see page 196).

- **Scrunching a towel or picking up marbles with your toes.** This is one of the best exercises there is for strengthening your arches and for keeping your plantar tendon healthy.

- **Roll the sole of your foot over a golf ball.** You can do this one while working at your desk, watching TV, or eating at the dinner table. Don't be shy about putting some good pressure into it. When your feet are healthy there will be very little, if any, pain. But if you're holding any tension in the soles of your feet, you'll definitely feel some productive discomfort.

- **Foot and ankle massage.** This is a great thing to do with a friend anytime. Katherine and I regularly trade foot massages, and it's one of the best things for relaxing your whole body . . . and for keeping your partner happy!

- **Spread your toes** anytime you find yourself without shoes on. It strengthens the muscles in your forefeet and arches, and improves circulation to your feet.

- **Plantar stretch.** Sit on your heels with your toes on the ground and your feet dorsiflexed.

- **Ankle stretch.** Sit on your calves with your knees on the ground and your toes pointed.

- **Walk or run barefoot.** This is a great way to strengthen and loosen all of the muscles and tendons in your feet. If you're not used to going barefoot, follow the principle of Gradual Progress and do it for only a few minutes at a time, gradually building up to more minutes. This might sound strange, but it's much better to run or walk on a *hard* surface, as this will allow your feet to educate the movement of your upper body.
- **Dorsiflex if you are sitting** for an extended period of time (at your desk or anywhere else). Point your toes toward your knee as often as you can remember to do so. It'll be much less tender when you get up to walk and it will stretch your calves and Achilles tendon.

For more information about injuries, visit our library of articles at www.chirunning.com.

Peak Performance and Race-Specific Training

Trying to do well and trying to beat others are two different things. Excellence and victory are conceptually distinct . . . and are experienced differently. —ALFIE KOHN

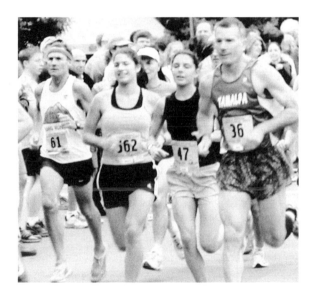

Most people think that a peak performance just happens, created by some invisible power. Sometimes it does happen that way—by grace. But you can have these experiences on a regular basis in your running, your racing, and your life if you set up the right conditions. It doesn't need to be a haphazard occurrence.

Peak performance is not about racing. It's about having a clear vision of how you'd like to improve yourself, setting a goal that embodies the vision, learning and practicing, and training your body to move in the direction of your vision. When the time is right, throwing yourself into a single event is a means to acknowledge what you've done and to learn what still needs some attention. A peak performance might be planned out over a six-month period, or it might happen spontaneously one day during a casual workout. It happens when you bring all that you are capable of into the activity before you and sustain it throughout. A peak performance isn't measured solely in results. It's measured internally *and* externally. It's how you feel before, during, and after an event, combined with the results.

When you have a peak performance, you're in harmony with what you are doing, and you're a conduit for the flow of chi. It's when you finish an event knowing that you've given it your best shot, doing all you were capable of. In these terms, a peak performance might not even be your fastest performance.

The venue for a peak performance is dictated by your level of conditioning and expertise. You wouldn't try for a peak performance on a 10K run if your goal is to run a good 5K. Likewise, you wouldn't go for a peak performance on a hilly course if you haven't done any hills in practice. A peak performance is when you accomplish what you have set out to do, and it is rarely an accident. It's intentional from the time you start your first training workout to the last stride of your event.

The key concept here is that you're striving for something beyond your current level of experience. You could be a first-time runner attempting to run a 12-minute mile or a seasoned runner aiming to finish your first marathon. It's all relative.

RACING

I love to race, mostly because it's the perfect opportunity to practice being present for an extended period of time. I love not only the race but also the training, planning, and strategizing. Racing, to me, is like a final exam to see how well I did my "homework" and whether or not all of my "studies" will pay off. A good day is when I finish well compared to my past performances. If I finish ahead of others in my age group, that's icing on the cake, but it's not the goal. I can have a peak performance no matter who finishes ahead of me.

Whenever I mention racing in my classes, people come back with statements like "I'm too old. I'm too slow." To which I respond that racing is the perfect opportunity to have a peak performance, and it could happen for anybody, at any level of skill or conditioning. You don't have to be a hotshot to have a peak performance. All it requires is that you put everything you know into what you are doing. Striving for a peak performance is an opportunity to see yourself really differently. It all comes back to setting up the right conditions for your energy to flow . . . and then magic happens.

"This is only a test." That familiar line lets us know that the radio in our dashboard will soon be emitting a screech that sounds like an owl in distress. But I like to use it to describe racing—it is only a test.

Performance anxiety brings up a lot of fears around racing. The best way to manage the associated stress is to eliminate it, which means studying your subject until it's as familiar as that face you see in the mirror each morning. This chapter is about how to train smart so you can run smart. Peak performance is not about muscle, it's about mind. It's about doing something well, with intention and finesse— doing the best you can do.

I'll use racing as a metaphor for preparing for a peak performance. Here's how I prepare for and run races so that I can create the conditions for a peak performance.

Here are the three main areas to pay attention to:

- **Your technique.** Have a good working knowledge of the ChiRunning focuses and how to apply them. Constantly work to perfect your technique, especially in the areas where you feel the weakest.
- **Your training.** Develop and plan a personally tailored program: daily, weekly, monthly. Have a good attitude about your program and exhibit perseverance with your training. Know what you need to do to get yourself from where you're starting to the day of your race in the best possible condition, physically and mentally.
- **Your event.** Have a clear logistical plan of what you intend to do on race day, along with a strategy for using everything that you have been practicing.

RACE-SPECIFIC TRAINING

I was always a lousy test taker in school. Aside from having poor study habits, I never learned how to figure out what would be required of me on test day. I had friends who seemed to barely study and ace every test. When I'd ask them how they did it, they would usually reply, "I just figured out what I thought they were going to ask and studied that. Then I just glossed over the rest." Easy for you to say.

The only real tests I take now are on race day. A race is a physical version of an exam. It's there to measure how well you prepared yourself and how well you work your way through all the problems that are presented. I *have* learned, from all my years of racing, how to do well on this type of test. This chapter is devoted to some of the tricks I've picked up along the way.

Whether you're a seasoned veteran of many races or it's your first race, you can optimize your chances of having a peak performance by doing some homework in the weeks leading up to the race.

It is not surprising that many races (those not large enough to attract the Kenyans) are won by locals. You can call it the home field advantage, but what does that mean in running? Quite simply, the locals get to practice on the course and familiarize themselves with all the nuances of the layout. They know when they can afford to rest, when to push the pace, and how to adjust their effort level with all of the little demands that the course will throw at them, because they've rehearsed their performance at the scene of the event. The smart runners know what to expect and train accordingly. Regardless of the distance, race-specific training gives you a huge advantage, whether you're trying to beat the competition or go for a personal best.

What is race-specific training? It's gearing your training toward as many of the specific challenges of an event as you can come up with, grouped into three categories: terrain, logistics, and personal experience. Training this way will prepare you better for anything that may come up on race day. Is the course hilly or flat? Will there be aid stations? Is it on trails, asphalt, or concrete? Will weather be a factor? Will the start be crowded? Answering these questions will give you a clearer sense of how to train yourself to be ready for *anything* when race day comes. Nobody likes to be blindsided, especially in a race.

A little planning goes a long way, but it's best to start your race-specific research a couple of months before the race. All race-specific training will be in *addition* to whatever you normally do to condition yourself.

Here are some suggestions for how to launch your race-specific training program.

- **Choose your distance.** What distance can you be well trained for when race day comes around? Be honest with yourself when assessing your current physical state. If you'd like to register for a race that is beyond your current conditioning level, be careful to give yourself plenty of time to get your mind and body up to speed before the event. If you train well for an event, it should not feel more difficult than any of your training runs.
- **Find an event.** Find a race within the parameters of what you'd *like* to train for. If you have a favorite area or type of terrain or environment that brings out the best in you, go for it. The choice is yours.
- **Learn about the course.** Many races have websites offering all the information you'll need. If it isn't in your vicinity, write or e-mail the race director for a map and an elevation profile. The most reliable resource for course information is to find people who have done the race in the past and pick their brain for all the details. The more people you can talk to, the more accurate your picture of the event will be. Drive the course if it's in your vicinity. Or better yet, run it. Then make notes of what the course is like, mile by mile.

Any good race-specific training program is designed around the answers to the following questions:

TERRAIN

- **What is the running surface like?** Does it change during the course? Do some of your training runs on the same type of surface.

I've met many runners who trained for a marathon on trails and then got hammered when they went to race a road marathon.

- **Are there any hills?** If so, how long and how steep are they? At what points in the race do the hills appear? Be sure to add hills at the same points they will occur in the race. Add hills to at least one of your weekly runs—preferably of the same height and grade—and/or substitute hill intervals for track workouts. If there is a significant hill 3 miles into a race, throw a significant hill 3 miles into your training runs. The goal of a successful hill runner is to hold a comfortable pace without getting tired legs. Be creative and design a racecourse mock-up in your area so you can go out and do weekly training runs on it.
- **What is the altitude of the course?** Is the altitude of the racecourse higher than where you normally train? If it's a significantly higher altitude, do some acclimation runs within two weeks of the actual race. If you don't live within driving distance of high-altitude running, you can help yourself out by practicing your belly-breathing technique during training runs to increase your oxygen intake. If the race is at a lower altitude, thank your lucky stars and have fun.

LOGISTICS

- **How often do aid stations appear,** and what will they be stocked with? Never eat or drink something in a race that you haven't tried out on your body beforehand. Who knows, you might be allergic to whatever sports drink they offer. If aid stations are too spread out for your needs, carry your own fluid supply. If you plan to drink the provided sports drink, try it during training runs to see if it works for you.
- **How big is the race?** Is it hundreds or thousands of people? If you're going for a personal best, don't pick a crowded race and make sure you start toward the front of the pack.
- **What time of day does the race start?** Within two weeks of the race date, begin most of your training runs at that time.
- **Will you be running with anyone else?** Will you be doing the whole race with friends, or maybe just starting the race with

friends? Be diligent about practicing *your* starting pace (slower than what you expect to average), and don't get swept into someone else's.

- **Have a start plan.** What is the first mile of the race like—flat, up-hill, or downhill? Start as many training runs as you can with a first mile similar to the first mile of the race. About two weeks before the race, practice starting slower than your projected average race pace. I mark off the first mile in quarter-mile increments with duct tape so that I can practice at my projected starting pace. In this way I can make small adjustments to my pace every quarter mile instead of running a mile and then realizing I'm way off pace. (I restrict my markings to roads—I never mark tracks or bike paths.)

PERSONAL EXPERIENCE

- **Have you run the distance?** It is a great physical and psychological advantage to run the race distance ahead of time so you know what your body will go through. Race day is not the best time to be going into frontierland.
- **How many weeks before the race?** Leave plenty of time to ramp up, train, and taper so you are in your best shape on race day. Two months before your race, adjust your regular training to include race-specific training.
- **Clean out your schedule for race week.** Do you have any other physical events close to the day of the race? Cancel them if this race means a lot to you. I've seen people ruin a race by doing something as innocent as gardening the day before. Plan to take off the two days before. If you're traveling there, get there early, set yourself up, and then chill.

GREAT TRAINING TIPS

Here are some more helpful guidelines for what to do during your race-specific training.

- **Hydration.** Practice drinking water while running. Drink electrolyte replacement drinks before and during your workouts. This will help to replace the minerals that your body loses when you sweat. You should drink 2 to 4 ounces of water for each fifteen to twenty minutes of running or walking on your training runs and during the race itself. Hydrate well before and during the race. Drink 12 to 20 ounces of water at least two hours before the race.

If you have a watch with a countdown timer (which I highly recommend), set it to beep every ten minutes and take a sip every time it goes off, *no matter what*. It helps to carry a water bottle with an electrolyte replacement. This will also be a major factor in whether or not your legs cramp up on you.

When I run a marathon distance or longer I always carry a water bottle in a waist pack. Here's why. At most marathons the aid stations are usually set every 2 miles. (You'll rarely see a marathon with water every mile.) That means that if I were a 10-minute-per-mile runner, I'd be getting a drink of water every twenty minutes at best. If this is the case, I run the risk of getting progressively dehydrated over the course of the four to six hours it might take me to finish the 26.2 miles. If I carry my water belt with me, I can hydrate every ten minutes and never get thirsty or dehydrated. This prevents me from having to be dependent on the aid stations to regulate my water intake. If you wait too long (twenty minutes or more) to drink water, you'll have a tendency to guzzle water when you finally see it, and then you're running with a bloated stomach. This could put you at risk of hyponatremia, a very dangerous situation where your body is losing salts from sweating and you're not replacing the electrolytes fast enough to keep a good salt balance in your system. When the salt content in your blood gets too low from taking in too much water and not enough electrolytes, your brain will start to malfunction, and then you're in big trouble. People have died from this. The best protection from hyponatremia is to drink small amounts of water regularly and take electrolyte replacements regularly.

- **Electrolyte replacement.** Whenever you're training for an event that is 10K or longer, it is highly recommended that you take some form of electrolyte replacement to make up for the loss of body salts due to perspiration. If the salt content of your body gets too low, your body won't be able to carry the tiny electrical impulses needed to fire your muscles, and you'll cramp. The two main electrolytes that need to be replaced are sodium and potassium. Sodium is found in most of your body fluids and concentrated in your blood, sweat, and tears. This is the salt you mainly lose when you sweat. Potassium can pass through cell membranes and provides electrolytes for the muscle cells. For this reason, you need both. So when you're shopping for an electrolyte replacement, whether it comes in powder, drink, or capsule form, look for one that contains both of these. The ingredient label should show a sodium/potassium ratio within a 3:1 to 5:1 range.

Electrolyte caps. Personally, I like to use electrolyte capsules. They're easy to use, don't take up a lot of room, aren't messy, and they keep the cramps away. If I'm in a race I simply tape them to my race bib with masking tape and swallow one every hour for the duration of the race. If it's a hot day, I'll take one every forty-five minutes. I've done this in races for years and never had leg cramps of any kind.

Electrolyte powders. If you prefer to carry your own powdered electrolyte replacement drink, you'll love this one (especially you ultra runners). Buy a couple of Gel Flasks (made by Ultimate Designs) at your local running store. They're small plastic pop-top bottles that hold only about 3 or 4 ounces. If you normally use a scoop of powder per 20-ounce water bottle you can get four bottles' worth of electrolyte replacement into each flask by mixing up a concentrated slurry of powder and warm water. Fill the flask halfway with water and pour in four scoops of powder (I mix mine with a chopstick). Keep your flask in your water belt. When you need a refill of electrolyte drink, just run through the next aid station with the top off your water bottle and ask a volunteer to pour water into it. When the bottle is near full, take out your handy-dandy flask and give it a squirt, and you're outta there in no time, with no sticky fingers.

Electrolyte drinks. Since I don't use electrolyte drinks, I can't honestly offer any recommendations. But I will give you this caution: there are very few electrolyte drinks that will replace electrolytes at the rate which you'll be losing them during an endurance event or a hot day. So, I would not depend solely on electrolyte replacement drinks during a marathon distance or longer.

- **Running and racing in extremely hot conditions.** If you're racing on a very hot day, check to see if the aid stations will have ice. Wear a hat with a brim, and if you can get ice, grab a few cubes and stick them in the top of your hat. You might need to tighten the brim so they won't fall out. As the ice slowly melts, it will keep your head cool, which, by the way, is crucial if you want to keep your brain working well. Heat exhaustion can strike when your brain's temperature rises even a small amount. If there isn't any ice available, soak a bandana and tie it on your head.

- **Fatigue.** There are a number of things you can do when you get tired on a run. Just because you're feeling tired doesn't necessarily mean you're at your physical limit. You could be doing something that is causing you to work harder than you need to.

I remember being at mile 80 in the Western States 100-Mile Endurance Run and feeling no energy left in my body. I wasn't sure how I was going to negotiate the last 20 miles, to make my goal of finishing in under twenty-four hours. I stopped at an aid station and picked up my pacer (in some ultras, you are allowed to have someone run with you after the halfway point), a runner whom I had been coaching for two years. She knew all the Form Focuses like the back of her hand and kept repeating them to me constantly all the way until the end of the race. Once I started engaging the focuses, I began to regain some of my mental and physical strength—enough, in fact, to make those last 20 miles the fastest of my entire race! Where did that energy come from? As I've said before, if you set up the right conditions, your chi will flow. As long as I had the strength to keep my form in good shape, I had the energy to run. Whenever I lapsed or lost my focus, I'd have to stop and walk, which was costing me valuable minutes. My pacer's mission was to keep my mind working by engaging me with focuses. When *that* was happening, I could keep myself running. Because of her constant reminders, I was able to finish a scant seven minutes ahead of my target time of twenty-four hours.

When you get tired, your form generally starts to fall apart, which in turn uses even more energy. It amazes me how much *more* tired I can get just thinking about how tired I *am*. On the other hand, it amazes me how much better I can feel when my body is aligned and relaxed. Here are some focuses to remember when you're feeling tired:

- Shorten your stride.
- Correct your posture. Make sure your feet are hitting behind your upper body, not in front of it.
- Engage your lean again, but don't bend at the waist.
- Slow down your pace until you recover some strength.
- Breathe more from your abdomen and increase your breath rate. Some people get tired from breathing too slowly.
- Don't focus on your fatigue, or you'll get more tired. Look up and take in the world around you.
- Relax your shoulders. Let your arms dangle at your sides for thirty seconds every 2 miles.
- Stay away from a shuffle. Pick up your heels and get your feet moving in a circular motion.

- **Race Diet** (for your regular training diet, see Chapter 11).

   Pre-race diet. Begin your pre-race diet six days before your race. Days six, five, and four before the race, eat protein for breakfast and dinner (soy products, meat, fish, or beans and rice). Days three, two, and one before the race, eat only carbohydrates (no protein), like whole wheat pasta (use meatless sauce), whole grains, and veggies.

   Race day diet. Eat foods that digest quickly, providing blood sugar. Eat lightly—bananas, toast and honey, fruits, dates or raisins—and don't eat anything you're not used to or anything that will still be in your stomach when you cross the finish line.

   Post-race diet. A good protein meal (meat, fish, poultry, tofu) helps your body rebuild muscle tissue. It's also important to replace minerals by eating leafy green salads and vegetables soon after the race. It is good to eat some form of carbohydrate after your race, but wait thirty minutes to two hours (depending on your digestive system). This will help to normalize your blood sugar levels and allow your body time to cool down significantly before ingesting food.

- **Starting pace.** When you are about a month away from race day, make an estimate of what you expect your average pace for the race will be. Then, for the four weeks preceding your event, practice your starting pace at least twice a week. Don't go out too fast! Most people start out too fast and burn out after a mile or two. Start at what you consider to be a comfortable, medium pace. Stay relaxed and you'll do much better.

  Go out and mark a 1-mile section of road that mimics the first mile of your race. Practice running a mile at a pace that's thirty seconds slower than your projected average pace per mile for the race. This will be your starting pace. Learn what it feels like in your body and remember it on race day.

- **Pre-race taper.** Taper off your training two weeks before the race, with no building or speed work. Don't do slower runs; just do shorter runs at the race pace. It's best to keep your legs sharp but rested.

- **Practice running hills.** If your race is hilly, train yourself by doing short hill intervals. These should be one to two minutes of uphill running followed by one to one and a half minutes of downhill. Start off easy and gradually build in intensity and speed with each interval. Be sure to warm up well before a hill workout. Do at least 2 miles of flat running before heading up. This will help to prevent muscle pulls due to cold muscles.

- **Train with a friend.** Find a training partner and use each other as inspiration to stay with your individual programs. You can also help each other by critiquing each other's running form.

- **Endurance training.** If you're training to do a 5K or 10K, build up to where you can run the distance at least once per week in training. You marathoners should be trained to run 26.2 miles on a moment's notice. Arthur Lydiard was legendary for his successful training of endurance runners. He would always have his athletes run far longer training runs than the actual event they were going to race. Training your body for endurance is the best guarantee that you'll have a good run on race day. If you want to build speed workouts into your training program, be sure to build a strong aerobic base *first*.

- **Asphalt running.** When you're out on your training runs, imagine yourself running on thin ice, and that will train you to run with a soft foot strike. If your race is on paved roads, do the majority of your training runs on pavement.
- **Shoes.** If you're planning to get new shoes for the race, buy and wear them at least three weeks before the race, not the same week! Most shoes tend to be stiff right out of the box, and you could get blisters from wearing shoes that aren't broken in yet.

RACE-DAY TIPS

Here's a list of reminders that will make your race day a positive and memorable event.

- **Arrive early.** Get yourself to the race with plenty of time for parking, walking to the start, and warming up with an easy jog.
- **Bring your alarm clock.** Set the countdown timer on your watch (if you have one) to beep *every ten minutes*. When it goes off, drink water and check in with your running focuses, especially your posture and lean.
- **Warm-up.** Start warming up twenty minutes before the race—jog at least one-half to 1 mile, depending on how much you feel your body needs. Do it at a very slow pace. Remember, you're just warming up your muscles and getting your circulation moving. Light stretching after you've warmed up can sometimes alleviate pre-race jitters. Do your Body Looseners. They'll give you something focused to do that will keep your mind more in the present. Check your shoes one more time to make sure your shoelaces are comfortable and won't come untied (tuck in the loops). Jog for ten minutes at an easy pace and then do some light stretches. After that, run a few light accelerations.

- **Go to the starting line.** Walk to where you plan to start and try to time it so you get there right before the gun goes off. You don't want to stand around letting your legs get stale. If you get there too early or the race has a late start, keep your legs moving. Shake them out, jog in place, walk around, do a few more strides.

- **Start off easy.** When the race starts, don't take off fast. Run easy for the first half mile. When you're running for one hour or more, you don't need to worry about losing a couple of minutes up front, and it could make the difference between simply completing the distance (or maybe not) and having a great race.

- **Check your pacing.** Check in with your pace at the first mile. If it's faster than your projected time, make an adjustment and slow yourself down. Relax and settle into a more reasonable pace. Don't say to yourself, "This pace doesn't feel that bad. I think I'll stay like this." You'll pay for it later. Check at the next mile marker to see if you've actually made the adjustment.

- **Check in with your preset splits.** Know beforehand approximately what time you want to be coming through your preset mile markers, and don't beat yourself up if you're behind a little—*caca pasa.*

- **Running form check-in.** Before the race, set your countdown timer to beep every ten minutes and be sure to start the timer soon after leaving the start line. *Every time* your beeper goes off, take a drink of water and check on your running form.

- **Drinking from paper cups at aid stations.** Have you ever grabbed a paper cup at an aid station in a race and spilled half of it before it reached your mouth? Try this. Grab the cup and, after thanking the volunteer who handed it to you, crimp the top so the only opening is a little spout between your thumb and forefinger. Hold the rest of the cup closed with your fingers and the heel of your hand and drink from the spout.

- **Make adjustments *before* you need to.** Drink *before* you're thirsty. Take in electrolytes *before* you cramp. Adjust your form before it starts to affect your running.

- **Additional, proven energy boosters.** Look up, smile, talk to someone, take in your surroundings, find someone ahead of you and try to "reel" him or her in, swing your arms more, check in with your focuses, smile some more.

- **Show gratitude.** Thank every race volunteer you see and cheer on every runner you pass.
- **Race recovery.** Cool down, stretch, do your leg drains, drink. When you get home, get into a hot bath ASAP.

While you're sitting in your hot bath, think about what you just did. How do you feel about the day? Did you do what you set out to do? Did you exceed your expectations? Basically, do an end-of-run review, and no matter what, acknowledge to yourself the positives that came from the experience. If there is anything you would do differently, take it as a lesson learned and turn it into a focus for future training runs.

Then massage your legs, drink more water, and eat a good solid protein meal. You deserve it!

On the day after your race, ride your bike or walk to loosen up your legs.

The success of your race will be directly proportional to the amount of planning and preparation that you put into it, on all levels. Some of these tips are to improve your physical advantage, and some are to improve your psychological advantage. Preparing yourself will help you to race your best and ace that test.

For Triathletes

Even some of the best-trained triathletes who are good runners seem to dread the run leg. You get off your bike and your legs feel like lead. It's like one of my recurring nightmares, where I'm running through knee-deep mud. Coming up to T-2 with little left in your legs can be somewhat unnerving if you're dependent on your legs to get you through the run. In answer to this dilemma, here are some helpful suggestions for turning that third leg into something to look forward to.

Focus on the right things (alignment, breathing fully, balance, technique, race strategy) and relax everything else, mentally and physically.

- **Start your run early.** Use the bike leg to prepare your legs for the run. When you have about 400 meters left to ride, change to *only pulling up on the pedals.* This will begin to fire your hip flexors and obliques, so when you get off the bike your legs will be set up to lift your ankles and pick up your feet instead of having to push you forward in your run.
- **Transition your legs.** When you get off the bike, shake out your legs and let them relax. You can even walk for a brief period before you begin running.
- **Let gravity do the work.** Run with a lean and *let gravity pull you forward.* There's your propulsion! Let your legs relax as much as possible between strides. Pick up your feet instead of pushing with your legs.
- **Gradual Progress.** Start your run leg with easy short strides and stay in first or second gear until your legs normalize to running.
- **Use a midfoot strike.** Feel your midfoot landing with every stride.
- **Take your body through a Body Scan.** Use the run leg to progressively rest and *relax* all parts of your body.
  - **Neck:** After the bike leg do neck rolls and look around during the first part of your run.
  - **Shoulders:** keep your elbows low and swinging to the rear.
  - **Arms:** periodically dangle them for thirty seconds at your sides. Once they're rested, you can swing them more fully to help your legs rest.
  - **Quads:** keep your knees down and let your heels float up behind you with each stride.
  - **Legs:** use your lean for propulsion.
  - **Ankles:** keep your lower legs from overworking by relaxing your ankles during every phase of your stride.

When you can truly relax in all the areas mentioned above, you'll begin to feel your energy returning. Use the list above for learning to relax during your swim and bike legs and you'll begin to see ways you can relax there too. If you are interested in using the ChiRunning principles for your swimming, I highly recommend Total Immersion Swimming developed by Terry Laughlin. When you're relaxed in your movement you can actually gain energy from whatever undertaking you're engaged in, instead of ending up wasted. As Master Xu once said, "It's not who wins the race, it's who lives longer."

RUNNING A MARATHON

Running a marathon has become the new frontier for exploring one's physical, mental, and emotional capacities. More than a million Americans run a marathon or half marathon every year, and the numbers keep increasing. The marathon, however, is presented in most books and magazines as a challenge in which one must endure great pain and hardship. The language you'll find includes "terror," "wracked with aches and pains," "expect pain," "26 miles of running hell," "like an auto accident," "your worst nightmare," and "the 26-mile monster."

In my ultramarathon training and in my racing career, I have run the marathon distance at least four hundred times. That sounds like I'm one of those fanatics. But my point is that I have experienced doing this without great hardship, and I know you can too. In the early days I did have some knee problems and occasional bouts of plantar fasciitis, which I have long since resolved by learning to run correctly. But otherwise, I can honestly say that running a marathon does not have to be, nor should be the terrorizing ordeal portrayed by so many. Many of our clients have had completely wonderful experiences running a marathon using the ChiRunning method.

Danny,

I just completed the Carlsbad Marathon and felt absolutely great! I'm 64 years old (the fastest 64-year-old in the race, I might add) and have been running for 31 years. I've tracked my mileage: now over 27,000. But this was only my second full marathon.

A few months ago I bought your book and DVD and it has

changed my life (how's that for a cliché?). I started applying the chi technique and at first it felt odd. In fact, my back and shoulders seemed to tighten up and I was about to discount the whole approach. Then I decided that maybe I was trying too hard and changing too much. Result: adjust back to tiny, incremental changes that led to a memorable 7-mile run down a canyon here in Utah—just relaxing.

I have worked on incorporating the technique for three months and am so impressed! At about mile 10 of the marathon, just as I was climbing a long hill, a spectator called out to me: "Nice form!" He must be a chi guy.

I had set my intention: to enjoy the marathon and feel good after. Man, I did exactly that . . . to a degree I never thought possible. I stayed relaxed and in form for the whole race and even had a kick at the end! About mile 22, I looked out over the Pacific and it was virtually a spiritual experience. I'll never forget the feeling.

I am totally converted to ChiRunning and looking forward to more marathons, halfs, and even a half Ironman Triathlon in June.

One more point, I have an absolute passion for encouraging and supporting senior-aged runners. I hope to run forever! Sixty-four is the new 46, and I'm living proof. Life is *good.* Thanks again for your work, your expertise, your clear instruction, and your encouragement.

All the best,

Paul R. Timm, Ph.D.

BTW, I went for runs of 4, 5, and 7 miles this week . . . all within days of completing the marathon. I cannot believe the ease of recovery. I'm virtually 100% ready to go at it again.

Running a marathon is an incredible challenge, not for enduring pain but for learning mastery over your physical and mental being. When you practice ChiRunning and train for a marathon in a mindful way, using the principle of Gradual Progress, you can learn to run a marathon in a way that is truly successful. ChiRunning offers an internal toolkit to overcome physical and emotional challenges and to provide the knowledge and confidence that gets you to the finish line in wonderful spirits and with a supple, relaxed, and healthy body. Pain, anguish, nightmares, and injury need no longer be an expected part of the marathon equation.

Here are the keys to success: Focus on form first. Then practice that form and deepen your understanding of it over longer distances. Build that distance slowly and safely until you can comfortably run the 26.2-mile distance. If it takes a year, then give yourself a year. If you learn the ChiRunning form easily and can already run a marathon or half marathon, you may be ready in three to six months. What matters most is that you do not hurt your body for the duration of your running life. What you will find is that the marathon is not an end unto itself, but is an opportunity to practice and develop qualities that increase the meaning and value of everyday life.

We have a ChiRunning Marathon Training program on our website at www.chirunning.com. We also have training programs for the half marathon, 10K, and 5K.

Peak performances and racing are opportunities to bring all your training and all your knowledge into an event. They can be wonderful challenges and very exhilarating. You should always allow yourself to fully enjoy your successes. At the same time, it's helpful to realize it is all a learning experience, and that the true meaning of success is not winning or losing but how you respond to each situation and how you choose to take the next step.

CHAPTER ELEVEN

Getting the Most Chi from Your Food

The wisdom of life consists in the elimination of non-essentials. —Lin Yu-tang

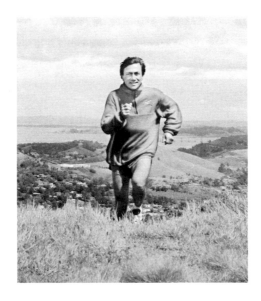

My belief is that your diet plays as important a role in your running as in your training. That's a pretty bold statement, but I will also say that all of us could improve our running by improving our diet, and there is no way you will reach your potential in running without at some point addressing the issue of fueling. If your diet is high-octane and clean, you'll gain access to greater amounts of chi, which will provide the necessary fuel for higher levels of performance.

I don't know about you, but diet has never been an easy subject for me. The trouble probably started when I was a kid. With three other siblings, dinner was a free-for-all. No matter how many people sat down to eat, there always seemed to be only enough food for that number minus one. If I wanted a full meal, I had to dive in with everyone else, or I might be left with crumbs. Some of that early experience still has a hold on my eating behavior today; I can still eat like there's not going to be enough food. I've worked against that tendency since I first articulated it to myself more than twenty-five years ago. I've gotten much better with it, but it still gets me sometimes. When I approach a meal in a relaxed and centered state, then I can slow down and enjoy the food, the company, and the experience. If I'm uptight, rushed, or just plain lazy, I can fall back into my former state quicker than a blink, and before I know it, I'm stuffed from overeating.

My issues with diet have, over the years, led me into the study and practice of getting the most from the food I eat. I've been blessed with some great teachers along the way and what I have found is that, as with ChiRunning, I need to set up the right conditions with my diet in order for chi to flow. This approach to diet has worked well for me for many years and will provide you with the guidelines for creating your own healthy diet. It's based on the accumulation of chi, which is really what eating should be all about. When your chi is flowing—whether from a good run or from fresh, wholesome food—you get deeply nourished. Let's take a look at how to set up the right conditions.

PRINCIPLES OF CHIRUNNING APPLIED TO DIET

There is so much information, and even conflicting information, about diet out there that it's hard to know which advice will work best for you. What has helped me most has been keeping myself on a diet plan based on the ChiRunning principles. Now, you're probably thinking, "Yeah, right. Let's hear Diet Plan No. 10,005." But hear me out, because these are sensible guidelines that are helpful no matter what your current approach to diet is, whether you're a vegetarian or an omnivore. These principles each shed light on an aspect of diet in a wholesome way.

NEEDLE IN COTTON

Gather to your center and let go of all else. In other words, being mindful of your diet is the first step in learning to let go of the foods and eating habits that no longer serve your running or your health. If you want your diet to have a positive and long-lasting effect on your life, you must stay with your intentions and remember why you're doing it.

I love cheese. I could eat it every day, lots of it, but it wreaks havoc on my body. When I eat too much of it, my head gets stuffy and I start to feel like a slug. So I limit myself to having cheese four times a week, because that's how much I can eat without my body feeling weird. As the principle says, gather to your center (my intentions around weekly cheese amounts) and let go of all else (the other times during the week that I crave cheese). Stick to your plan—*that's* gathering to your center. And don't be drawn off track by all the things that will pull you off center and away from your plan. Anytime you gather to your center, you gather chi and build inner strength.

GRADUAL PROGRESS:
THE STEP-BY-STEP APPROACH

If you want to eat a cleaner, more wholesome diet—which I recommend—then allow yourself, and your body, some time to develop new habits relative to food. Don't expect yourself to be great at your diet right away. It's not an easy subject to deal with, so take small but progressive steps to achieve your goals. Make small changes and let them be cumulative. It's just like learning the ChiRunning focuses, which come more easily if you practice one at a time. When it's really in your system, you can add another brick to the foundation. Take your time and do it right. You'll build more chi by being solid within each step along the way.

For example, if you want to reduce your sugar intake (which I highly recommend as well), don't try to do it while you're also trying to cut back on caffeine and you have an intense project due at work in a few weeks. Just work on eliminating sugar, and when you're solid with that, begin to reduce your caffeine intake.

The amount of inner strength (chi) gained by improving one small aspect of your diet will give you the confidence to take on additional improvements. Rest assured that the cumulative effect of changing many aspects of your diet for the better will be transformative.

BALANCE

In order to maintain strong chi in your system, it is important to keep a balance among the nutrients necessary for your body to run well. My average seems to be 60 to 70% carbohydrates, 15 to 20% proteins, and 20 to 25% fats. You need to figure out what works for you. These are three food groups that need to be in balance to fuel your body in the healthiest way. If your nutritional balance is out of whack, your available energy will fluctuate instead of being a nice steady burn. This will result in mood swings, peaks and valleys in your energy, and a certain level of unpredictability in your life in general.

High-quality foods = high-quality energy. In addition to eating this proportional balance, it's also important that the carbohydrates, proteins, and fats are the highest quality. If you eat a high-quality diet, your body will be balanced in two ways: it will be nutritionally balanced with the right proportions of the three food groups, and it will also be balanced relative to the energy demands of an active life.

There are many things that will throw the body into a state of imbalance. Too many sweets, too much protein, and fried foods of any kind are a few examples. Our society seems driven by sweets and desserts. Sugar is in everything, especially processed foods, so it's easy to eat too many quick-burning sugars that send your blood sugar through the roof and then let you down with the subtlety of an auctioneer's gavel. The all-American diet also seems to contain some form of meat at least once a day; that's way more animal protein than your body needs. And our culture is hooked on saturated fats, which come mainly in the form of fried foods, processed cooking oils, butter, and animal products. A little bit is fine, but the amount that most people eat is out of balance with our bodies' real needs.

Another aspect of balance high on the list of anyone trying to regulate weight is between calories eaten and calories burned. If you want to lose weight, the balance has to swing toward burning more calories than you take in. If you'd like to gain weight, you'll need to eat more calories than you burn. It's a very simple formula that has dictated body proportions since the age of cavemen, and it's a great example of applied thermodynamics.

THE PYRAMID

The pyramid applies to your diet by suggesting that you have a very strong foundation in foods that deliver the most chi with the least amount of energy required to process them. As we go up the pyramid, we find foods that we still need in our diet, but in lesser amounts, and with the awareness that more of these foods is not better; they need to be consumed in proportion to the base of the pyramid.

This pyramid is not the official USDA food pyramid. It's based on the diet I've been enjoying with great results for more than twenty years. Once again, these are general guidelines. If you are a vegetarian or an endurance athlete, modify this pyramid for your needs.

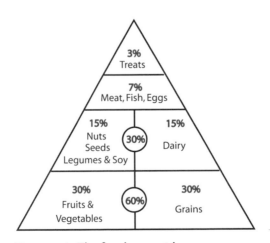

Figure 126—The food pyramid

- **Level 1.** In order for you to have a healthy, clean-burning fuel supply, the foundation of your diet (the base of your pyramid) should be made up of grains, fruits, and vegetables. Not only are fruits and vegetables a good source of clean-burning carbohydrate fuel, they also provide your body with much-needed antioxidants, which are free-radical scavengers. Free radicals in your cell tissues are produced by exercise and take much of the blame for everything from cancer to depletion of the immune system and premature aging. Whole grains are underappreciated and underutilized in our culture. They are slow-burning complex carbohydrates that provide a steady, long-term source of energy. When whole grains are processed and refined, they become fast-burning, simple carbohydrates and low-octane fuel. My favorite whole-grain foods are brown rice, kasha (buckwheat groats), oats, cornmeal, bulgur, and whole wheat bread. Fully 60% of my diet comes from Level I of the pyramid—30% from fruits and vegetables and 30% from whole grains.

- **Level 2.** The next level of foods makes up 30% of my diet: 15% from nuts, seeds, and legumes (soy products, nut butters, dried beans, and lentils) and 15% from dairy (cheese, yogurt, and milk). If you're not into dairy, you'll need to make up for your lack of fat and protein with plant-based products. But if you *are* into dairy, keep it to only 15% of your diet. You need Level 2 foods in your diet in order to maintain strong chi in your system, but the quantity (30%) is half the amount of Level 1.

- **Level 3.** In my diet, the third level consists of meat, fish, and eggs, which I eat regularly but sparingly. It makes up a total of 7% of what I eat. I have fish once a week, meat or tofu once a week, and eggs one to two times a week. When animal protein is overconsumed, it depletes chi because of the intense processing it requires. When you do eat meat, it should be the highest quality possible, and organic when available. If you're a vegetarian, you'll get protein from plant-based sources, such as legumes, and fats from oils, nuts, and nut butters.

- **Level 4.** Three percent of your diet should be from foods that are not necessarily eaten for nutritional reasons but are nourishing on other levels. I eat a yummy dessert once or twice a week, but when I'm tempted to eat too many sweets, I remind myself that I get more pleasure from having lots of chi than I do from being buzzed on sweets. There's no doubt about it—too much sugar depletes your immune system and can quickly throw a solid pyramid out of balance. Caffeine falls into this group. Although it has been proven to enhance mental alertness and improve performance, it is also a diuretic that increases water loss. So if you mix caffeine with running, take it with plenty of water.

The following foods are not doing you any favors nutritionally and are not a part of the pyramid: candy, commercial condiments, processed foods, preservatives, additives, white flour (including bagels and most pastas), refined sugar, and sodas. These foods deplete your energy, and it's best to use them as little as possible or get them out of your diet altogether.

The pyramid serves as a visual reminder of where our strength really comes from, and shows the relative importance of certain types of foods in our lives. Be aware that this pyramid is designed for an *active* lifestyle, not a sedentary one.

Non-Identification: Getting Yourself Out of the Way

Non-identification is really what maintaining a good diet is all about. We get stuck on ideas about ourselves and our diet that are not based on a true understanding of what our body needs. Anytime you're stuck on an idea about your weight or your diet, you're "identified," meaning you are using your ego and not Body Sensing to guide your decisions. Examples: "I'm addicted to chocolate," "I can't get going in the morning without my coffee," "I have to have meat every day or I won't have the strength I need," "I need bread at lunch or I'll still be hungry." Non-identification with your diet means that in order to best support your current level of activity, you eat what you *need*, not what you *want*.

Non-identification means you're acting totally in the best interests of your body. Imagine what it's like to be in a good place with your diet—to make strong, healthy decisions and be able to see them through.

The number one way to learn about your real needs is to Body Sense. The proof of good diet is measured over time. How does your body feel immediately after eating? Six hours later? The next day? Ask yourself and listen closely to your body's responses. It will tell you if you're on the right track or not.

PRACTICAL STEPS FOR A HEALTHY DIET

One of the most profound things I have learned from studying healthy lifestyles is how important diet is in our lives. As I attempt to live more holistically, I am led to look at my diet in the same way I would any other activity—with a view to its part in the larger scheme of my life. I need to pay attention not only to *what* I eat but also to *how much* I eat, *when* I eat, and *how* I eat.

WHAT TO EAT

If you want high-quality runs, *eat high-quality foods*. If your body isn't being supported by a good diet, it's like buying a Ferrari and putting low-octane gas in the tank. You can get much higher performance out of a car if it's running on premium fuel. It's as simple as that.

Whenever you sit down to a meal, think about where the food came from and whether you think it has a lot of life and energy still in it. There is no question that the most beautiful area of the grocery store is the produce section. There's a reason for that—the foods there have more life in them. Organic foods, including meat and dairy, are cleaner and closer to Nature than those that have been grown with chemical fertilizers and pesticides. I'm not going to give you specifics of what to eat (that's a whole 'nother book), but I do want you to start thinking about what you put in your mouth and why.

HIGH-CHI FOODS

- Organic foods
- Fresh foods
- Freshly prepared foods
- Locally grown foods

LOW-CHI OR NO-CHI FOODS

- Most canned foods
- Overcooked foods
- Processed and refined foods
- Fried foods
- Microwaved foods
- Foods with additives, preservatives, or coloring
- Pickled foods
- Condiments (commercially produced)
- Smoked foods
- Most restaurant foods, especially fast-food venues

A great teacher set me up with my diet plan, and I am eternally grateful for having had this window into the power of a well-designed diet. Here's an overview.

I eat two main meals a day. I eat a hearty meal every morning. Three times a week it's a big bowl of hot whole-grain cereal loaded with nuts, seeds, and dried fruit. Once a week it's a substantial egg meal, and twice a week it's a bowl of grain and vegetables with nuts and sometimes cheese. Once a week I have yogurt with lots of nuts, seeds, raisins, and fruit. At midday I eat a light lunch, which might include dried fruit with nuts, fresh fruit with cheese, or tea and crackers.

My weekly dinner menu looks something like this: a meat meal once a month, fish once a week, a huge salad once a week, and beans and rice once a week. On the other nights I have grain-and-vegetable meals, sometimes with nuts, seeds, and/or cheese or tofu.

I always get the freshest organic ingredients available, and they are worth the extra cost. The meals are simple, delicious, and wonderfully satisfying.

WHEN TO EAT

Your body will work much better if your refueling is done in a cyclical manner. Eat your meals at the same times every day. This allows your stomach to work more efficiently, because the cycles of digestion are consistent in duration. Eating between meals makes your stomach work harder to digest freshly eaten food on top of food that is already in process—double duty. I eat my breakfast and dinner approximately twelve hours apart, because that's roughly the amount of time it takes for my stomach to completely digest a meal. I have a light lunch at midday, and if I need an energy boost during the late morning or afternoon, I'll have a cup of tea with honey (refined sugar spikes my blood sugar).

TIMING IS EVERYTHING

Not only is the quality of your food important but, as they say, timing is everything. Your body will have different nutritional needs depending on your workout schedule. If you've just done a strenuous workout, one of your next two meals should be a solid protein meal to rebuild your muscles. It's also good to get in a hearty salad to put valuable minerals back into your system. By planning your meals ahead of time, you can match what is happening in your training schedule.

The basic rule of thumb is to eat a carbohydrate meal before a hard workout and a protein meal after. If you run in the morning, do your fueling the evening before. This allows you to get up, get dressed, and head out the door. A heavy meal the night before a hard workout might not be fully digested by the time you go out to run, which will slow you down considerably. High-octane, quick-burning fuel will help your workout to go much better.

If you eat before you run, be sure it's at least three hours prior. If you do have to eat before running, a banana helps your blood sugar level and is a good source of potassium.

HOW TO EAT

To get the most chi out of your food, a few things will need to be in order. Your environment at mealtime has much to do with the quality of the chi you gain from the meal. At mealtime you should settle down to take in nourishment and replenish your energy stores. The key to ensuring a high-quality meal is stillness.

Transitioning into a meal is the best way to get off to a nourishing start. First, make your eating environment a clear and settling space. Light a candle or decorate the eating area with a small flower arrangement. Remove any semblance of chaos. Make sure you have everything you need for your meal before you sit down so you don't have to get up once you've started eating.

Take a little time to remember what you're doing—you're taking in nourishment. As in your running, start off slowly. The beginning of the meal sets the pace for how it unfolds. If you start off too fast, the whole meal will be fast, and you'll finish with a full belly and still not feel nourished. Your food will not be well chewed, your stomach will have to work harder to digest it in its rough state, and you'll most likely feel like a toad when you get up from the table, instead of vibrant and replenished. Eat slowly and take small bites. (Do I sound like your mother yet?) Sit up straight and remember to breathe between bites.

Eating well and with a true respect for our bodies and the foods we eat is paramount to having a healthy body and maintaining a high-quality lifestyle.

Running and Weight Loss

Yes, you can lose weight through running, but here's the deal. Weight management is a product of calories in and calories out. The best way to regulate your weight is with a wise combination of diet *and* running. If you want to gain weight, eat more calories than you expend. If you want to lose weight, eat fewer calories than you expend. It's the law, and there is no way around it.

Don't let the job of maintaining a healthy weight fall solely on the shoulders of your running. One of the problems with that is when you can't run (because of injury, travel, etc.), you have nothing to fall back on to maintain your weight. My best advice: if you want to regulate your weight, learn to regulate your diet first, and let your running regulate your toning.

One way to regulate your weight through running is to use your long runs to burn fat calories. It is a myth that you lose weight by doing shorter, faster (glycogen-burning) workouts. When you run at a comfortable aerobic pace for longer than thirty minutes your body burns less glycogen and more fat calories. This means that, as long as you don't increase the amount of food you eat, you're directly reducing the amount of fat in your body.

Just as grains and vegetables are the foundation of a healthy diet, a good diet is the foundation for a successful running program and a vibrant life. I can't stress enough the importance of diet. The whole idea here is to put into your mouth only that which will deeply nourish you. Eating well *really* matters.

Recommended Reading

These books on diet, nutrition, and natural health are some of the best and most thorough knowledge available, in my opinion.

Dynamic Nutrition for Maximum Performance, by Daniel Gastelu and Dr. Fred Hatfield, Avery Publishing Group, 1997.

The Encyclopedia of Natural Medicine (2nd ed.), by Michael Murray, N.D., and Joseph Pizzorno, N.D., Prima Publishing, 1998.

Smart Medicine for Healthier Living, by Janet Zand, L.Ac., O.M.D., Allan N. Spreen, M.D., C.N.C., and James B. LaValle, R.Ph., N.D., Avery Publishing Group, 1999.

Between Heaven and Earth: A Guide to Chinese Medicine, by Harriet Beinfield, L.Ac., and Efrem Korngold, L.Ac., O.M.D., Ballantine Books, 1991.

Feeding the Whole Family, by Cynthia Lair, Moon Smile Press, 1997.

CHAPTER TWELVE

Run as You Live, Live as You Run

There is a life-force within your soul, seek that life.
There is a gem in the mountain of your body, seek that mine.
O traveler, if you are in search of That
Don't look outside, look inside yourself and seek That. —RUMI

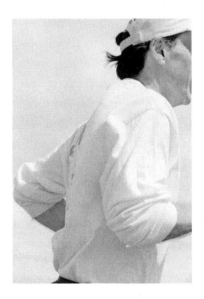

I just got back from my Sunday cruise run, and I feel like a new person. My week was way busier than normal, and I needed to get out of the house and into the hills. I arrived at the trailhead feeling a bit groggy from writing until all hours the night before, and I was really looking forward to the run because I *knew* I would return to my car feeling better than when I left. Indeed, I was able to totally turn my energy around within two hours. In the past, it might have taken days or weeks. There are a few personal activities I have to thank for that: a consistent running program, a high-quality diet, a meditation practice, sufficient rest, and a keen awareness that letting up on any one of the above is not an option.

I lived in a very small, close-knit neighborhood with neighbors who'd knock on your door when it started to rain and tell you your car windows were down. Marge lived across the street. We considered her the village elder, because she cared so much about all the families up and down the block. What I most appreciated about her was her attitude toward life. When I'd see her out in her garden watering the plants, I'd usually ask how she was doing, to which she inevitably replied, with a twinkle in her eye, "I've got a lot to be thankful for . . . I woke up today. And when you get to be my age, things like that are important." I couldn't have agreed more on both counts. She was a model for me of someone who took advantage of every day, because she knew that she might not be around the next day. She was fit as a fiddle and sharp as a tack because she had spent years eating well, exercising, caring for others, and generally holding the attitude that life is something to be treasured every day.

Our culture offers little in terms of training us how to live and appreciate life from the inside out. So much of our focus is on the external that little attention is put on feeling what goes on internally. I'm not suggesting we should all be isolationists or self-centered. I'm saying that we can all best contribute to society if we first and foremost sense and acknowledge our own feelings, then act from a sense of who we really are, not from an idea of what will earn us the most positive responses or avoid the most negative ones.

How does one get to this elusive place of centeredness? Of all the principles discussed in Chapter 2, the most important is Needle in Cotton. Whenever you go out for a run, practice this principle, and it will guide you to be centered in your running and in your life. Needle in Cotton is infused within all the ChiRunning themes—planning, staying relaxed, breathing, working with balance in mind, taking small steps to ensure Gradual Progress, practicing Non-identification in the face of challenges and setbacks, and building a strong base that is unshakable in its support for your actions. By consistently using these themes in your ChiRunning program, you'll begin to see how they apply in your life.

I have a client who tells me that whenever she comes up against a situation in which she feels at a loss, she asks herself, "If this were a run, how would I approach the solution, and what adjustment would I make?" She says it never fails to help her find the answer inside her own body of knowledge. Here's a letter she sent recently:

> Danny,
> I think the real benefit of ChiRunning is not only being able to run without pain but applying the ideas to all aspects of my life. I am now working on trying to use the "form" to help me live my life more freely and easily, free from stress and other types of pain (e.g., emotional, intellectual). I am seeing that the same principles that are used to make running less of an effort and more efficient can be used to help my life be more calm and peaceful in a world that seems crazy and chaotic at times. If I can try to relax when I feel tired or overwhelmed, or if I return to my center when I feel stress or anxiety, then I will have truly adopted the principles of ChiRunning. From a purely physical viewpoint, ChiRunning can be used to run faster and farther and will definitely make me a better and more relaxed runner. However, I feel that there is so much more to it than that. By practicing the principles of Body Sensing and efficiently using my muscle energy to enjoy my runs, it teaches me that I can learn to sense myself physically and emotionally in all situations and to not waste energy as I journey through life. I know that incorporating this philosophy with a holistic focus will enable me to achieve a true sense of peace and happiness.
>
> Aga Goodsell

For me, the practice of ChiRunning helps maintain a clear, strong sense of connection with my body—which translates, in no uncertain terms, to inner freedom: The freedom to not be intimidated by challenges I face. The freedom to follow my intuition instead of second-guessing my choices. The freedom to allow my present condition to guide my future but not rule it.

This sense of freedom is what makes it possible to live life creatively. My wife always tells me that she doesn't consider herself a creative person. She compares herself to the artists and creative people she has surrounded herself with her entire life, but she doesn't feel that she's in their league. Quite the contrary, I see her as being highly creative, not only in how she lives her life but also in being who she is. She is rock-solid in her beliefs and holds to them, knowing they are based in Truth. She creates her own life every day by embodying her beliefs and knowledge of what's best. She's not driven by the goals of others, and I rarely see her going along with the general trends of our culture without deeply questioning their benefits and drawbacks. She holds to her center and meets her challenges with the grace of a T'ai Chi master. And she is taking the utmost care in creatively passing on that knowledge to our daughter.

Creativity has many forms, and it's my assertion that we can all be creative beings if we can learn to center our lives with programs that allow us to experience ourselves being grounded in our bodies. Embodying the Needle in Cotton principle allows you to be driven by what is inside of *you*, not by what is inside of someone else.

T'ai Chi is based on the principle of Needle in Cotton, which means moving and living from one's center. It's a theme that we could all use in our approach to this fast-paced world. Things might not always fall exactly how you'd like them to. But when you're centered, you can be creative and fluid in responding to anything that happens.

Master Xu says that whenever he fights an opponent in training, he has no idea what is going to happen, because it's a creative act. He told me about an incident that happened just after he moved to this country from China. He was walking home from the grocery store when a gang of six guys (some with knives) surrounded him on the street and demanded money. When he refused to give it to them, they came in for the attack. *Big* mistake. The next thing he remembers is that all of them were lying on the ground around him; one had to be taken to the hospital. He said his body just took over and responded in an instant to everything that was coming at him. There was no thought process involved; it was a purely creative act. I experience a similar type of creativity when I'm running down a single-track trail at high speed. I get into an inner zone of stillness while rocks and trees come at me in a blur of motion. I watch my body do the running while I sit back and enjoy the ride. That's when running feels more like dancing than danger.

How to turn what you learn from ChiRunning into useful everyday habits would fill a book by itself (which will happen when we write *ChiLiving*). The easiest way to transfer all of this information to your life in general is to go back and read this book from the start, and every time you see the words *run* and *running,* just substitute *live* and *living.* Watch how they work interchangeably.

GUIDELINES FOR CHILIVING

Use the Chi-Skills from Chapter 3 when approaching everything from a business project to grocery shopping. Practice them all the time. The best way to begin transferring your ChiRunning knowledge into the rest of your life is to start each day with the Body Scan exercise from Chapter 3. Do it consistently, every day if possible. Use it to get in touch with your body first thing in the morning. Believe me, it's better for you than a cup of coffee: It launches you into the morning conscious of your body instead of your head. Later in the day, when you're sitting in your car or at your desk, return to Body Sensing and do another Body Scan. If you sense any tension or discomfort, you can soften that area and move on. Do little remembrances like this all day long—sensing and correcting, making adjustments as you go. When your posture isn't straight, make an adjustment. When you find yourself not breathing, make an adjustment. If you find yourself holding tension somewhere, relax it. If you want to build a center, practice bringing your attention to the spine all day long.

Make your workday a moving meditation in which you constantly bring attention to your spine. Focusing on your spine and your breathing are two centering devices that have been used in meditation practices for centuries. Sitting in meditation, one focuses on keeping the spine still, which then positions movement as its complement. In this way one learns to accommodate stillness in the midst of activity. Remembering your spine and your breath brings you into the present moment, from which many possibilities of action can spring forth.

When you're running, keeping your posture in line brings you to your center. When you're *not* running, the same thing applies.

OPENING NEW DOORS

A little over three years ago, Eddie started running. He had grown up in Manhattan, and the only time he ever ran was when he was late for the A train. His brother needed a kidney transplant, so Eddie took up running to get himself into the physical shape needed to be a healthy donor. He never ended up having to donate his kidney, thankfully, but it got him started. He subsequently moved to California and ran more often, and within a year he found himself running his first marathon. The second year, after taking a series of ChiRunning classes, he ran five marathons; this past year he ran eight marathons, three 50Ks (31.1 miles each), a 50-miler, and a 100K (62 miles). If he keeps it up at this rate, I figure he should be able to run to Hawaii sometime next year.

What makes Eddie's story remarkable is that he is 56 years old. More than anything, it has been his attitude that has allowed him to run these distances without being intimidated by them.

He has practiced the focuses since his first ChiRunning class six years ago, and they have become a great set of tools that he uses in every run. Now, whenever he meets a challenging section of a run, he knows that there is always something he can do to help himself through it. When I asked him what goes through his head when he considers running longer and longer distances, he told me that all he had to do was the required preparation—which for him meant consistent training and enjoyment of the process.

He has an incredibly infectious positive attitude, which I believe frees him to do what he needs to do without wasting energy worrying about how it's going to get done or what the outcome will be. When I asked him to sum up his attitude about running, he said, "Any day that you don't finish a run is still a day that you went out for a beautiful run. If that's the downside, then there's no downside!"

ChiRunning leaves you with a sense of confidence that if you approach anything with a realistic vision, a well-thought-out plan, and a consistent, step-by-step approach, you can accomplish great things.

It's about doing the necessary work of maintaining and carefully building your base so that growth—albeit slow sometimes—is always in a forward direction. When you feel centered in yourself, with the confidence that years of mindful living produce, you are freed up to live your life creatively while keeping to your practice. You are externally consistent with the actions that allow you to live a rich life while staying internally free. It's all about enjoying the process of growth and not being overfocused on results.

As you become increasingly familiar with the Chi-Skills, you will begin to open windows and doors to levels of experience that you never dreamed possible. Seeing each level and finding new sets of possibilities there is like taking the elevator up in a skycraper and checking out the view every ten stories. Each new vista is quite different. What seemed larger than life from the ground floor looks much smaller and less significant when you are looking down at it from the upper stories. When you get to the top of the building, you notice that the city is really surrounded by miles of open space and places to explore.

Creative running, or creative living, means developing your skills to the point where you're not intimidated by anything thrown at you. As the ChiRunning skills become more integrated into your regular routine, living an extraordinary life will seem normal.

Appendix

A GUIDE TO THE MUSCLES REFERRED TO IN THE BOOK

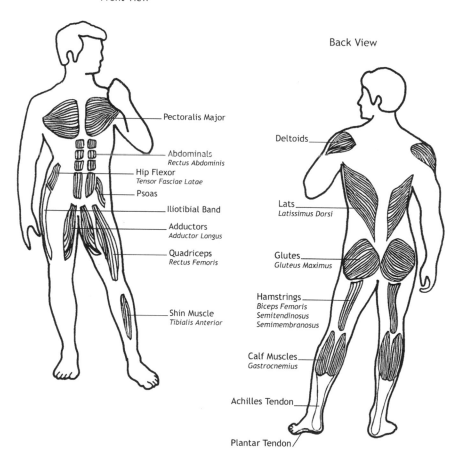

Front View

Pectoralis Major

Abdominals
Rectus Abdominis

Hip Flexor
Tensor Fasciae Latae

Psoas

Iliotibial Band

Adductors
Adductor Longus

Quadriceps
Rectus Femoris

Shin Muscle
Tibialis Anterior

Back View

Deltoids

Lats
Latissimus Dorsi

Glutes
Gluteus Maximus

Hamstrings
Biceps Femoris
Semitendinosus
Semimembranosus

Calf Muscles
Gastrocnemius

Achilles Tendon

Plantar Tendon

Acknowledgments

Katherine and I would like to pay tribute to the following people for their support in this work. Some have helped us directly and some indirectly, but all have played important roles. I can't imagine playing on a better team.

Master Xu, we will be indebted to you forever for teaching us how to bring chi into our lives. Your generosity with transmitting ancient Chinese wisdom into the simple act of running fills us with deep respect.

A huge thanks to all the Certified ChiRunning and ChiWalking Instructors. Your dedication and input has been invaluable. A special thanks to Chris Griffin and Kathy Griest, two of our most dedicated Master Instructors. To all the students of ChiRunning, this book is the result of everything you taught us. Thank you also for your feedback, suggestions, and encouragement, which were always timely. Thank you, Jim Dunn, for adding plenty of spice to our lives. My gratitude goes out to Aga Goodsell. Thanks for all those miles together. You are the perfect model for the book because the form is so in your body.

Terry Laughlin, Total Immersion Swimming and ChiRunning are like twin sons of different mothers and we appreciate how you have led the way in the trend of intelligent movement. It is mind-boggling how closely Total Immersion Swimming and ChiRunning are aligned at their core levels.

Dr. Mark Cucuzzella, your selfless efforts to bring the message of ChiRunning into the medical community are deeply appreciated. Your own success as a runner is a living testimonial to sound biomechanics combined with a pure joy of running.

Ryan Miller, no wonder you're so fast. You're as close to pure spirit as anyone we've ever known.

Bonnie Solow, our angel book agent, your guidance throughout this process has been such a blessing. Zach Schisgal, it's a pleasure working with a truly great editor. Lori Cheung, your photography stands the test of time. Your contribution has been giant. Frank Veronsky, loved working with you on the cover shot. A special thanks goes out to Chris Lloreda, Shida, Cherlynne, and all you very special folks at Simon & Schuster for your enthusiasm and help.

Many thanks to our larger community of friends and foes, running partners, competitors, and all those who have brought out our best by offering challenge and support.

Mei Ling, you walked into our lives out of nowhere and have become the ultimate running and walking companion. Your enthusiasm for running is unsurpassed.

We'd like to pay tribute to our parents and siblings whose support and encouragement have been essential.

And finally to our daughter, Journey. You are the inspiration behind all that we do.

Index